A Survivor's Journey

BEATING
OVARIAN
CANCER

*How to Overcome the Odds
and Reclaim Your Life*

CHRIS BLEDY

AVIVA
PUBLISHING
NEW YORK

Beating Ovarian Cancer
How to Overcome the Odds and Reclaim Your Life

Published by:
Aviva Publishing
2301 Saranac Avenue, Ste. 100
Lake Placid, NY 12946
518-523-1320
www.avivapubs.com

Printed in the United States of America

Library of Congress Control Number: 2008929882

ISBN: 978-1-890427-67-2

Acknowledgements

I must thank my lifelong friend Michele Michaels, who kept at me for years about writing this book. When I was too sick to write, she spent hours documenting my thoughts on cassette tapes. Without her vision, assistance and motivation, this book would not be possible.

And to my friend Dolby Dubrow, who not only encouraged me to write this book, but instilled me with belief that my story is worth telling.

My deepest gratitude goes to Richard L. Friedman, MD for his significant and valuable contributions to this book, and to my life. More than anything else, I am thankful for his years of care and expertise.

I'm so appreciative to John L. Barstis, MD for sharing his excitement about the future of effective treatments and for providing important information on current chemotherapy options for ovarian cancer patients.

Special thanks go to Hulda Regehr Clark, PhD, ND, for her tireless dedication, ongoing scientific research and numerous publications on curing cancer. Her bravery in the face of ridicule and mockery is as astounding as her cure rates.

I am honored and grateful to Rick Evans for creating the artwork in this book. Rick is well known for his lifetime devotion and amazing talent in airbrush art.

Many people contributed to this book, but none participated more in my healing than my family; my greatest fortune. It's my family I want to thank the most.

My husband Les; the protector, provider, lover and comedian; he dedicated years toward my healing. He is wonderfully powerful and he used his chi to pull me from death's doorstep more than once. There aren't enough words to describe my love for him.

My mother, my children, my grandsons, my sisters, my brother, my nieces, my nephews, my cousins, my in-laws and my entire extended family all deserve my sincerest thanks and deepest appreciation. Their love and support was unyielding. There was never a time when I felt unloved or uncared for, all because of this incredible family of mine. I love you all.

I am privileged in having a genuinely loving family, true friends and close acquaintances. Although there is not enough room to name each individually, you know who you are and more importantly, I know who you are. I treasure each of you and thank you from the bottom of my heart.

Dedication

This book is dedicated to each of you whose lives have been touched in some way by ovarian cancer. It is for those fighting the disease and for those living with it. It is written in memory of all women taken by ovarian cancer, and for those who battled beside me, who I miss and think of often.

Contents

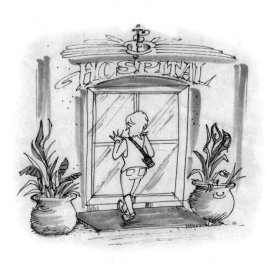

The Down and Dirty

In January 2000, I was diagnosed with advanced ovarian cancer. I had my first cancer operation on Valentine's Day. After five hours of surgery, I was sent to the Intensive Care Unit for four days and then I spent four days in a private room on the cancer floor.

I'd not only had a complete hysterectomy with plenty of lymph nodes removed, I had a far more radical procedure. I awoke with a temporary colostomy and catheter. The lower part of my colon and the upper part of my rectum had been removed. My ureter was rebuilt and then re-implanted into my bladder. The cancer had been severe throughout my pelvic area. They told me I'd have the colostomy for six months and the catheter for two weeks.

While a colostomy bag is hidden from view, it's almost impossible to hide a catheter. It's one thing to have a "pee bag" hanging off the side of your hospital bed; carrying it around like a purse is another. At first, I thought it wouldn't be so bad since it would only be two weeks and I'd just be staying at home. But it wasn't that simple. Clothes were an issue. Underwear was out of the question and so were pants. Apparently, staying out of public view was also out of the question. I had to go to an office building for chemo, to the hospital for an IVP (an x-ray to look at my urinary system) and cystogram (another x-ray to check my urinary system) and to the doctor's office to have the catheter removed. None of these places have private entrances. Even though I felt like I was the walking dead, I tried to keep my sense of humor. So, for the next two weeks, I referred to my pee bag as my new purse. And I simply couldn't go anywhere without my new purse!

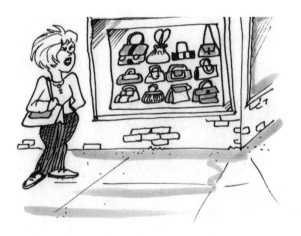

Three days after being released from the hospital, I began standard doses of chemotherapy (Taxol and Carboplatin) for six months. Chemo was complete hell for me. Although I wasn't thrilled about having "second-look" surgery, I did look forward to having my colostomy reversed. In fact, I'd never spent so much time living in the future, just waiting to get rid of that bag and the burdensome details that went along with it.

My second-look surgery was in July and it was no party, I can assure you. Again, I was cut from pubic bone to breast bone. The colostomy reversal was a success and more than one hundred biopsies proved I was cancer free!

The only problem was that I just didn't feel right. I figured it must be from having been cut open again. You know, follow the dotted line, same scar as my first surgery. For some reason, it didn't feel right, though. I couldn't bend or move properly. The pain hurt deep inside the pit of my stomach and I quietly wondered if the surgeon had left an instrument inside me during the second-look surgery. After all, I had been through this surgery only six months ago and hadn't experienced this type of discomfort then.

My insides hurt and the colostomy reversal resulted in my having to spend endless time on the toilet. This time, recovery was tougher than I expected. I don't know why I'd thought it would be easier the second time around. After all, it was still major surgery, so perhaps my body just needed some extra time. I remained patient and upbeat. Surely, things were looking up for me. The chemo treatments were over, the colostomy was gone and my hair was even returning! I reminded myself often that everything takes time. Some things just take more time than others.

About sixteen weeks later, I developed a tender bump near my belly button on my incision scar. The incision had healed up nicely, but now I had a flaming red sore spot there. On Halloween, it started bleeding and I ended up in the doctor's office. To make a long story short, they'd used a different type of suture material during my second-look surgery. As it turned out, the problem was with Panacryl, a highly touted, new suture material recently approved by the FDA. This began my long nightmare, about a two-year nightmare in fact.

My body was unable to dissolve the internal sutures, so I developed boil-like bumps that finally opened and bled. They were like wormholes, where the suture material worked its way out of my body. Now, I'd always liked the idea of wormholes and time travel, but this certainly wasn't what I had in mind. This was awful. I had to pack these "wormholes" with Sorbsan (a cotton-like material) using the wooden end of a long cotton swab.

Then after weeks, sometimes months, of packing a hole, the suture material finally emerged. My doctor pulled out as much as I could tolerate and then he cut it. I'm usually very tough about pain, but tears and screams were not unusual with this. My tolerance for pain wore dreadfully thin. The wormholes continued to appear all along my incision and it got to the point where I looked like I had six or seven belly buttons. They lined up above and below my true belly button. I felt as if the entire center of my being was being wrenched. It took effort to stand upright and not to stand hunched over. Just when I thought the suture ordeal was over, another bump appeared. It seemed an endless ordeal.

I asked my surgeon what was behind the decision to use Panacryl suture material for my second-look surgery. He said, "The risk of hernias in midline incisions is around ten or fifteen percent. Our hope was that improving the suture material would reduce your long-term risk of developing hernias." Unfortunately, the Panacryl caused more hell than I can describe.

There were a lot of problems associated with Panacryl. It was recalled in March 2006 because it didn't dissolve in the body as intended. I can't help but wonder why it took so long for this recall. I'm sure I wasn't the only person who called Ethicon, Panacryl's manufacturer, to complain about this defective product all those years ago. Their pathetic response about how my doctor must not have been properly trained in suturing techniques disgusts me. Now after all these years, Ethicon finally has to admit the truth. I cannot begin to explain the amount of agony and suffering I endured because of that product.

Even with these issues, two years after my second-look surgery, I truly believed I had beaten cancer. I had done everything the doctors prescribed and went faithfully for my check-ups every twelve weeks. Then in May 2002, my doctor discovered a swollen lymph node in my neck.

Out came a syringe. The doctor took a biopsy and immediately sent it off to the lab for results. A few days later, I learned that my cancer was back. Even though I no longer had ovaries, these were the same type of ovarian cancer cells – and now they had reappeared in my neck.

I was upset and very angry. After everything I had been through, it just didn't seem possible. And it didn't seem fair. I couldn't comprehend it. I just couldn't have cancer again. Not me. No way.

I went into denial. For the past two years, even with all the crap I'd been through, I'd remained always positive, always upbeat. I had done things so thoughtfully, always taking the high road, always looking for the positive. No, this simply could not be happening.

For the next few weeks, I went through just about every emotion you can imagine. I procrastinated about having another surgery and more chemo. I'd do anything to avoid having chemo again. That was the one thing I didn't think I could tolerate another time.

Chemo. It never gets easier. It's cumulative. Each treatment gets worse. Two days after receiving a chemo treatment, I could count on being in bed for one solid week. I could barely raise my head. I felt like I was going to pass out when I tried to sit up or walk. It was like having a horrible case of the flu or something worse. I just wanted to bury my head under the covers until it all went away. I remember lying on the floor alone, crying. My insides felt like creepy crawlers were taking over. I couldn't think straight. I couldn't read, watch TV or focus on anything. I was bald – and I mean completely hairless – ugly and very sick. I just wanted to die. No, I didn't think I could do chemo again.

From the time I'd been first diagnosed with cancer in 2000, until the time of my recurrence in 2002, I had toyed with alternative and complementary treatments. I'd read books on different ways to fight cancer without surgery, chemotherapy or radiation. I'll admit I hadn't really done anything seriously. A little here and a little there was about it. After all, I thought I was cured. Now, I had to face the cancer demon again.

The problem with ovarian cancer is that it's extremely difficult to cure once it reaches the late stages. And unfortunately, most women with ovarian cancer are diagnosed in the late stages. There is no early detection test and symptoms are practically non-existent. This is why it's known as "The Silent Killer." Some say it whispers. Yet, even when a woman hears the whispers and seeks treatment, she is usually misdiagnosed or disregarded completely. It's a very tough disease to diagnose and even tougher to cure.

Ovarian cancer is now treated as a chronic disease. In other words, it keeps coming back. This means a lifetime of surgeries and a variety of chemotherapy drugs. Your doctor's goal becomes to manage the disease. In other words, you just keep getting treatments until treatment no longer works. How lucky could I get? Not only did I get advanced ovarian cancer, but I also got a recurring chronic disease.

Since my diagnosis, I've learned more than I ever wanted to know about cancer. I hadn't known anything about ovarian cancer except that Gilda Radner had died from the disease. I'd thought ovarian cancer could be detected with a Pap test. I was wrong. My Pap test had been normal, even though I had full-blown ovarian cancer.

Now my cancer was back and I had to make decisions. What to do? What could I do? I felt so hopeless and out of control. At that point, other people held my fate in their hands. I was at the mercy of doctors and traditional medicine. I felt out of control. It was then that I decided to try some alternatives to conventional medicine. I know it might sound radical, but what could be more radical than going under the knife again and enduring more chemotherapy?

For the next couple of months, I participated in extensive alternative treatments. In fact, I spent two weeks in Mexico under the care of Dr. Hulda Clark, author of *The Cure for All*

Advanced Cancers. Her treatments involve identifying and eliminating various parasites and toxic substances found in my diseased body. I received education about nutrition, supplements, killing parasites, mercury in dental work, creating safe surroundings and much more. I'd learned that this type of personal care isn't available here in the U.S. It was frustrating to find so many obstacles to any path that deviates from conventional medicine.

We are not as free as we think we are. When it comes to medical treatment, we don't have freedom of choice. When I was diagnosed with cancer, the only treatment offered was surgery and chemotherapy – nothing else. It is practically impossible to find alternative care in the United States. Even when traditional treatment has failed, we're still not allowed to obtain alternative treatments. While *information* about alternative treatments is abundant and easily accessible here in the U.S., the challenge is in having it *administered.* You must administer the treatment yourself or leave the country to get personal care. It is sad, but true. So, I did as many others have done and left the country to get treated.

Most people can't afford to leave their jobs, go to another country and pay for medical treatment out of their own pockets. Since I could only afford two weeks of treatment in Mexico, I learned as much as possible before and during that time and continued the treatments at home for many weeks afterwards.

I felt that I was cured, and if not cured, I was well on my way to being cured. I still had to deal with my surgeon, though. He wanted to do a third surgery and for good reasons, too. Before I left the country (which I didn't discuss with him), I had a PET scan. My doctor wanted to deal with some questionable spots on the scan and he wanted to remove the cancerous lymph node in my neck.

While those were his motives, my motives for surgery were different. I wanted to get rid of any of the remaining Panacryl suture material that had haunted me for the past two years.

My doctor reassured me that he would clean out the Panacryl and would use fast-dissolving suture materials. In fact, he surprised me and said that he would also get rid of the many dimples along my incision (I called them extra belly buttons). So, he'd be cleaning up my scar as well. That was welcome news. Of course, I'd still have the scar, but not the deep indentations from those "wormholes." So there I was, agreeing to another surgery. In fact, I was curious about what he would find once he opened me up. For me, it might also be a good indicator as to whether the alternative treatments were having a positive impact on my health.

After my third operation, the news was inconclusive. My doctor had been very aggressive with all my surgeries and this one was to be no different. Since I was young and healthy, he was willing to take some risks in order to assure the best possible outcome. Once again, he cleaned out the cancer with meticulous care. Not only were there positive lymph nodes in my neck to be removed, but there was also an issue with my pancreas. During surgery, my doctor called in a colleague for another opinion. Between the two of them, they simply couldn't determine what was going on with my pancreas. At first, they thought it might be pancreatic cancer, but they couldn't be sure. There were cancerous lymph nodes around and under my pancreas, but that didn't answer the question of whether or not I had pancreatic cancer. They took a biopsy of my pancreas and removed the cancerous lymph nodes.

After surgery, the surgeon delivered the news to my husband. Because they hadn't received the biopsy results yet, the surgeon outlined all the possibilities. If it was pancreatic cancer, then I only had a few weeks to live. It could be ovarian cancer on the pancreas or it could be pancreatitis. They really didn't know what it was just yet.

It turned out to be chronic pancreatitis. Another chronic condition! Wasn't it enough to have chronic ovarian cancer? Now I had chronic pancreatitis, too. I have to admit that I completely ignored the diagnosis of chronic pancreatitis. After all, I had recurring ovarian cancer. And let's face it; I'd known too many people with ovarian cancer. Once the recurrences started, these women all went quickly. There was no talk of the cancer appearing anywhere else.

I wondered about my pancreas, though. I'd thought chronic pancreatitis was something alcoholics got after years of excessive drinking. I'd never been much of a drinker, so I knew that wasn't the cause with me. Could I have somehow developed this condition in only two years? After all, I'd had two major surgeries in 2000 and I didn't have chronic pancreatitis then. Maybe there had been cancer on my pancreas and now it was something else. Perhaps it had changed because of my recent alternative treatments. It's highly doubtful, but nothing is impossible. I guess I'll never know how much my alternative treatments impacted my cancer at that time. After all, I only did the alternative treatments for about three months. Still, I wonder if it might be possible that some alternative treatments really do work, or, at the very least, help.

There was so much to think about. I was grateful for this last surgery for several reasons. One was the relief I felt knowing the torturous Panacryl ordeal was finally over. I could tell it was gone, too. That underlying stress vanished. I was very grateful for the removal of the cancerous lymph nodes and the additional information provided by this last surgery. I don't have pancreatic cancer or any other cancer. I didn't know what my alternative treatments had accomplished, but I believe that what I did had a positive impact on my health in a short time.

As I thought about this, I continued to research alternative and complementary therapies. I tried new and different approaches. I stuck to what was safe and healthy. I like to keep things as simple and natural as possible. I learned many things and tried so much. It was fun and frustrating at the same time. I shared what I was doing with friends and family, but rarely with any medical professionals. I didn't want to be discouraged or taken lightly. Mostly, I kept the information and what I was doing to myself. I didn't even try to share it with my doctor. Physicians in the U.S. can't go on the record in support of your participation in alternative or complementary treatments. They could lose their license to practice medicine by doing so, and I realize that.

I have tremendous admiration, respect and gratitude for my doctor. I adore him in many ways. My cancer was extremely advanced and I know that each of my surgeries was necessary. I believe with all my heart that my doctor literally saved my life. In my opinion, he's the best there is and I am forever grateful for his care. Not only that, he is a wonderful person, too. He always gives hugs, encouragement and love.

It is important to realize that this book is not about snubbing conventional medicine; it is about actively participating in your own treatment and recovery. This book is about taking care of yourself once treatments are completed.

During any type of cancer treatment, the patient receives a lot of attention, direction and instruction. But once treatment is complete, we don't know what to do. We live in fear of recurrences; counting down the days, hoping to reach the magic five-year marker. We wonder if we've been cured or if we are simply in remission.

Please realize that your doctors can't cure you; they can only provide treatment. The healing and curing is up to you. Your doctor may be able to treat your burned hand, but if you continually place your hand in the fire, there really isn't much any doctor can do for you. It's your responsibility to keep your hand out of the fire, and no amount of treatment will change that.

On my follow-up visit with my surgeon, the topic of chemotherapy came up again. I'd had such an internal battle with this topic. I said, "No." He said, "Yes." I understood my doctor's concern. He truly believed chemotherapy was the best attack. I disagreed, only because I just couldn't face it again. The memories were too close to the surface and too raw. First, I absolutely refused to go back to my previous oncologist. Next, he suggested a different oncologist. I reluctantly agreed to a consultation. When all was said and done, my insurance company wouldn't approve that particular oncologist. I was relieved for a couple reasons. One, I didn't want to go through the standard chemotherapy treatment again, and two, it was a welcomed delay.

After months of bantering back and forth, I got a referral to another oncologist. This doctor wasn't nearby, but he's a UCLA medical oncologist who knows a lot about ovarian cancer. I told him exactly how I felt about chemotherapy, stressing that I would rather die than go through chemo again. This doctor understood completely. He knew exactly what I had gone through. We discussed different treatment options. He talked me into a weekly low-dose treatment of Taxol and Carboplatin and assured me it would be much easier to tolerate and just as effective. He promised that I could stop at once, at any time, if I wasn't satisfied. Although I didn't want to go through it again, pressure from my family, friends and my surgeon was too much, so I agreed to give it a try. I was angry about having to go through chemo again, but I got over it. However, I was more committed than ever to stick with my natural and complementary treatments.

Anything other than conventional medicine is considered complementary treatment. It's important to understand the differences in the terms *alternative* and *complementary*. Alternative treatments are used *instead of* conventional treatments. Complementary treatments are used *in addition to* conventional treatments. A growing number of people prefer to use the more contemporary term *integrative* medicine. Integrative medicine includes traditional, alternative and complementary therapies. Since I've used them all, I suppose the term *integrative* applies best in my situation.

Many people use complementary therapies during their traditional treatment. I wasn't one of those people. I used my complementary therapies after completing my conventional treatments. I didn't want to take any unnecessary risks and I didn't want to muddy the waters with a mixture of treatments. I wanted to get through the conventional treatment so I could get on with the crucial work of rebuilding my new body, inside and out. I looked at it as though I'd be starting with a clean slate. I could go back to doing what I'd done before and probably get the same results (cancer again), or I could do things differently and possibly avoid cancer completely.

I had a new mission: Staying healthy, vibrantly healthy. That's a big mission for someone with chronic ovarian cancer and chronic pancreatitis. Since chronic seemed to be a key word with me, I decided to shoot for *chronic* fabulous health!

Although there isn't much that can be done for chronic pancreatitis, I found that taking digestive enzymes and keeping to a healthy diet helps tremendously.

As I mentioned earlier, recurring ovarian cancer is also considered a chronic disease. The pattern is that each remission gets shorter and shorter. You keep getting treatment until you no longer respond. Since my recurrence took place about two years after I'd been declared cancer free, my cancer was expected to return in less than two years.

Well, the cancer has not returned! It's been more than five years since my recurrence and my results are better than ever. People who know me are amazed and I think my doctors are, too.

It seems that everyone knows someone who has cancer. People always ask me what I've done to stay healthy. How did I get to this point? What integrative therapies do I use? What do I recommend? I get phone calls from people I don't even know. They get my number through The Wellness Community or through friends, family or acquaintances. People are searching for alternatives and complementary treatments. I know I was searching – and I still am. I continually try new things and adjust my life program. A few staples always remain, but change is part of life and as my life changes, so does my life program. New discoveries and information are always available, so there's always something new to try.

As you can tell by my brief history, I do not recommend that you ignore or replace traditional treatments. I am quick to refer women to my gynecologic oncologist whenever there are suspicious female problems. I am not a doctor and I make no medical claims in this book. I present this as information only. Consider it a testimony to the actions I took during my journey with cancer. Each of us is different and the things we choose will be different. This book reflects my very personal viewpoint – and my very personal story. I certainly have not been exposed to all available treatments and I'll admit to being biased in my presentation. This is how I approached my ovarian cancer and my personal health.

I realize there is no known "cure" for cancer, no real breakthrough or headline news telling us a cure has been discovered. Still, thousands of people have won the battle. How did they do it? Is it possible that you and I can win this challenge and beat the odds? I think it is indeed possible.

Please understand, I am just a regular person out here. I am fighting a disease, as are so many others. I don't get any special treatments, deals or discounts for any of the products or services mentioned in this book. I am not endorsing or promoting anything. These are just personal choices I've made. I buy these things just like you do or I get them passed on to me from friends or family. It's all been trial and error, so to speak. I will talk about things that have helped me or that have worked for me personally. If this information or any of these products can help anyone else, then I am blessed to pass them on.

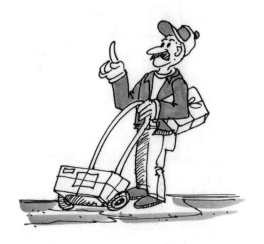

You've Got Cancer

I don't care what type of cancer you have; when you receive that diagnosis, it is devastating news. Hearing those words, "You've got cancer," is like having your death certificate handed to you right then and there. My sister Carlyn once told me that any time she hears that someone has cancer, her heart aches because she knows that whether the person lives or dies, it's going to be one rough journey. I thought about this and about what my sister said one day as I was listening to an old Bob Dylan tune, "A Hard Rain's A-Gonna Fall." It sure did fall for me.

I didn't know what to do or how to react. I was shocked, to be certain. I never expected it to be cancer. Menopause, yes, but cancer wasn't even on my radar. I felt like I had been delivered the wrong package. The package was addressed to me, but I didn't want it. The worst part was – I couldn't return it. For me, I'd never even known anyone close who'd had cancer. It didn't run in my family, but maybe that was because so many in my family had died young from heart disease. Again, I am reminded that the only reason I'd even heard of ovarian cancer was because of Gilda Radner. At the time, I'd thought she was probably too busy to have her regular exams. I didn't know that there is no early detection test for ovarian cancer. There was a lot I didn't know about this disease. Well, actually I didn't know anything!

Naturally, I first broke the news to my husband, Les. The words somehow came out. "They think I have ovarian cancer, but they won't say for sure. I'm being referred to a specialist; a gynecologic oncologist." Boy, did I cry. My poor husband...I know he must have been freaked out. We were in our late forties and too young to be going through this. Les was strong and protective. He lovingly reassured me that everything was going to be fine. Somehow, we'd get through this. He reminded me, "They really don't know for sure, so let's wait and see what this specialist says."

I met my gynecologic oncologist, Richard L. Friedman, MD, on Friday, February 4, 2000. I think I was his last appointment for the day. The office was quiet as I sat alone and anxiety-ridden in the waiting room. This kind man actually came out to the waiting room, took me by the hand and led me to his office. We talked for quite some time. I was practically in tears as I explained all the exams and tests I'd had and how no one had really told me anything. Well, all that changed. Dr. Friedman told me everything about the tests, his concerns and more. Then he said that he was going to examine me and he stressed that the only opinion that counted was his. From now on, I would be under his care and I wasn't to worry about anything that had happened prior to my visit with him. He was so genuine and sincere. I finally felt like I was exactly where I was supposed to be. I was under the care of a compassionate specialist.

After my exam, we looked at his calendar and immediately scheduled a surgery date. He wanted to do the surgery as soon as possible. Oh yeah, this was serious. He informed me of the various possible outcomes from surgery, including a temporary colostomy. Again, I was shocked. This was very grave, yet I still knew very little about my disease. Everything had happened so quickly. I sensed the urgency all around me. I'd barely had time to absorb the fact that I had cancer, let alone all this other stuff. Now I had about ten days to decide who to tell and what to tell them.

There were family, friends, adults and children. And the job…oh yeah, work. Where should I start? Maybe this isn't a big deal to you, but for many women, these issues *are* a big deal. Many women don't want everyone to know they have ovarian cancer. There are a variety reasons for this. Some women feel they will be treated differently. Others have personal issues with certain family members or acquaintances. It could be anything from the patient's age to wanting to prevent additional stress on someone who is already ill. Whatever the reason, not everyone handles the news in the same way.

My husband and I decided it was best to come out with it and let everyone know. Ours is a close family. That's just the way we are. It doesn't matter if we see each other every day or if it's been weeks or months, the love is always there. I am lucky to have this. No matter how you do it, though, telling people about your disease is an extremely emotional experience. We kept it brief, explaining my diagnosis of ovarian cancer, the scheduled surgery and chemo to follow. There were lots of tears, fears and questions. It wasn't easy for me, but I'm sure it was hell for the rest of them. Naturally, we told only the adults and left the decision about informing the children to their parents. Since our children were all adults, I didn't have the concerns of small children in the home. I cannot imagine the bravery it takes for young women to face those precious little faces with explanations of cancer.

As far as my job went, that was an easy one for me. I worked as a consultant, so there wouldn't be any leave of absence or sick pay. I've known my employer, Nancy, for more than twenty years. We'd had a previous career together at the phone company. Because of our long relationship and the fact that she is a woman, it was easy to be honest with her. Again, I was lucky to have such wonderful people in my life. Just like that, my working days ended for several years to come.

Thank God I had health insurance. You hear horror stories about HMOs and people often complain about the quality of care, but my HMO turned out to be great. That's not to say it was perfect. Authorizations were delayed a couple of times, but nothing that compromised my treatments. As you can see, I'm still here to talk about it. I know people who've had to sell their homes and spend their entire life savings just to have treatment. Surgery and chemo costs are off the charts! I don't know how women without insurance handle it. I used to complain about the high cost of my health insurance; the monthly premiums were more than my car payment. You won't hear me complain any more. In fact, I am grateful for the ability to make an insurance payment.

The reason I brought up HMOs is because so many people worry that if they have an HMO, then somehow their treatment will be substandard. I know my treatment was top-notch. My gynecologic oncologist is among the very best. Dr. Friedman is well-known and highly recognized in his field. I often speak with other patients in the waiting room; over and over I hear praise for this man. For many patients, he is the only doctor they will accept. This was quite reassuring for me since I was one of the patients who didn't have a choice. My HMO simply sent me there. The point is, don't freak out if you have an HMO. Even an HMO should be able to get you under the care of a gynecologic oncologist. If you have ovarian cancer or if your doctors suspect you have it, you should be referred immediately to a gynecologic oncologist. A regular gynecologist or medi-cal oncologist will not do – not for ovarian cancer. If you are not automatically referred as I was, you must insist on it. A gynecologic oncologist is the only person who should operate on you. It truly can mean the difference between life and death.

Hearing that you have cancer is terrifying. However, it doesn't mean you're being handed a death certificate. Yes, the treatment is tough. Yes, you will have to make some ad-justments in your life. No one says it will be easy, but it can be done. Cancer can be beaten. Even advanced ovarian can-cer has survivors. How come I'm doing so well? People ask me this question all the time. They want to know what I'm doing, especially women with recurring ovarian cancer.

So often, recurring ovarian cancer means shorter remis-sion times. The cancer comes back quicker each time. I've seen this with my own eyes on a very personal level. I've been to far too many funerals. I've lost too many friends and acquaintances to recurring ovarian cancer. I want to change that. Yes, I do want to survive, but I also want you to survive. Not just survive, but also live a healthy and fulfilling life. And I want you to feel good and look good. I want you to have a zest for life. And most important, I want you to regain control of your body, your mind and your health.

Believe me; I know this is not an easy goal, even for people who are healthy. When my cancer came back, it really hit me hard. I felt I was destined to die. I thought, "This really is it. This is how I'm going to die." Mentally, I revisited my demons over and over. I was angry and I hated cancer. I calculated how much time might remain for me. Was it a year – or two? What value should I put on that time? Would it be valuable? Was I going to die sick and ugly? How could I do this without being pathetic? Could I possibly find a way to make these years some of my best? If so, how? Could I rediscover love, joy, laughter and more? Did I want to? Maybe I should just go with everyone feeling sorry for me.

I decided, "To hell with it! Yes, I am going to die, but eventually, so is everyone else. If this is the end, then I want to be proud of it." That's what I set out to do, to end my life proudly. I wanted people to remember the real me, not the routine person created by my daily commitments and chores. Cancer or not, it's still me inside here.

I decided I was going to come out and live. I was going to end my years joyously and gratefully. The only way I could do that was to rebuild my strength as much as possible, little by little. I took it in small steps. If I could only do one pleasing thing that day, then that's what I did. Whatever it was, I did it and I felt gratitude. Every small thing I did made a small difference. Before you know it, small things add up. They add up in a big way.

No matter how easy, how small or how simple, never underestimate the power of your pleasing deeds. When I say pleasing, I mean pleasing to you. When you do something that is pleasing – be it physically, mentally or spiritually, you will benefit. The more you benefit, the more others benefit. One thing cancer patients know that others may not is the value of the present moment. The present moment is truly all any of us have. The past cannot be altered and the future, well the future simply isn't here. I say, "If all I have is this moment, then let it be grand."

Consider this part of your life's journey. There is much to learn and much that can be done. Your cancer doesn't affect just you; it affects all those around you, particularly those who love you. You are more treasured than you realize. Your survival means a great deal. Never doubt your value or your worthiness. There is so much to live for. Life is filled with joy, beauty and love. Sure, there are plenty of challenges, but the contrast is what makes life so fulfilling. I want to defeat this illness so I can continue to experience this great gift called life. For now, let's live and learn.

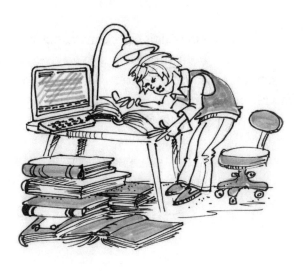

Ovarian Cancer

Here I was at the beginning of 2000, the new millennium, a year the entire world looked toward with great hope and anticipation. I was stuck at the computer looking at site after site about ovarian cancer. Wow. If you want to get educated easily and quickly, the Internet is the way to go. It's like information heaven. At first, it was exciting to have abundant resources at my fingertips. Day after day, I searched. I searched for cures, for clinical trials, for miracles, for anything that would make it better. I wanted to learn everything I could about ovarian cancer. I'll admit that at first, I was dazed and a bit overwhelmed at the amount of information available about treatments, surgeries, chemotherapies and more. But it was exactly what I wanted and needed to know. My knowledge of cancer was zero. I was "cancer ignorant." It was nice while it lasted.

One of the first things that struck me about cancer was the term "five-year survival rate." Why was five years considered such a big deal? I sat there in my forties, thinking five years meant nothing. I was wrong. Reaching the five-year marker is a big deal. It often means you've beaten the beast. Getting there is another thing. It becomes one more thing to obsess over. After treatment, you count the days and hope they become months then pray the months become years. The closer you get to the magic five-year mark, the slower the clock moves. Tick-tock, tick-tock. Then do you suddenly become free of fear once you've achieved this goal? Is it the end of cancer once and for all? The five-year marker doesn't seem to be as magical for ovarian cancer folks. Many live with the disease, rather than beat it. It made no difference which site I visited; the dreadful statistics varied only slightly. It was sad and scary. I spent hours online. I quickly became addicted.

While the Internet is loaded with information, including some inspirational personal sites, over time I found it depressed me. Instead of feeling better about being informed, I felt doomed and somewhat hopeless. I decided to stay away from the Internet for a while. It interfered with my normally upbeat perspective. I knew that I wanted and needed this knowledge, but how could I use it to my advantage? I hadn't even come to terms with my own emotions. Also, there were mounds of information to sort through.

If you have ovarian cancer, it's going to take time to accept it. Take heart. The emotional roller coaster does eventually come to an end. The anger, depression and fear take some time, though. Somehow, we all find a way to face it. Once I learned the important details about ovarian cancer, the facts and fiction, I realized that ovarian cancer could be managed. Actually, managing it may be a very good approach. Before you can manage anything, though, you need to have an understanding of exactly what you're attempting to manage. There is plenty to learn, so let's get on with the story.

Symptoms

My ovarian cancer was discovered during a visit to the gynecologist when I was forty-eight years old. I had always had regular periods, every twenty-eight days or so. Before that visit to the doctor, I had missed one period completely. The following month, I had my period on schedule, but two weeks later I had another period. I immediately made an appointment with my gynecologist. Naturally, I suspected menopause was knocking at the door. So, my discussion with the doctor centered on my going through menopause. My doctor agreed this was likely, given my age. Still, she wanted to do a complete exam.

During my pelvic exam, the doctor said she thought she felt something, perhaps a cyst or growth, but she couldn't be sure. She scheduled me for an ultrasound. After the ultrasound, I knew it would be a week or so before I heard the results, but I wasn't concerned. So when the call came, I was surprised because it was the doctor herself on the phone. She explained that the ultrasound showed a growth, in fact a very large growth. Still, she was optimistic and didn't want to frighten me. However, she did want me to come in immediately for a blood test, also to see another doctor. Since I felt absolutely normal, I really wasn't worried. I had just returned from a vacation in Hawaii. I played tennis regularly and kept up with my busy work schedule. I figured it was probably some type of benign growth that would have to be removed. Boy was I wrong. Apparently, ovarian cancer doesn't necessarily come with feelings of illness.

As I mentioned earlier, ovarian cancer is called "The Silent Killer." We know now that it isn't completely silent. It does "whisper." It whispers so softly, though, that often women feel as though they had no symptoms at all. Even when symptoms do appear, they may be so vague that they are ignored. Symptoms tend to be non-specific and can mimic other conditions such as irritable bowel syndrome or even aging.

Symptoms include:
- Increased abdominal size
- Bloating or discomfort
- Changes in bladder function
- Constipation or diarrhea
- Shortness of breath
- Fatigue
- Unusual weight gain or weight loss
- Vaginal bleeding
- Pain with intercourse
- [a] Pelvic pain

This is crazy! What woman doesn't complain about being bloated? Yes, I experienced fatigue, but what working woman doesn't? After all, most of us work all day, come home, make dinner and take care of our families. I was floored by the fact that these are the symptoms for ovarian cancer. Even if I'd gone to the doctor with these symptoms, do you really think anyone would have started off suspecting cancer? I think I would have been labeled as a complainer or hypochondriac. This was just too frustrating to even think about. But think about it I did.

Believe it or not, I learned that most women do experience some of these symptoms for more than six months prior to being diagnosed. Since many of the symptoms come with aging, it's easy to see how they can be ignored. I looked at the symptoms again and again. I wondered if I'd had any of the symptoms and simply dismissed them. I mean, the symptoms aren't particularly unique or alarming.

Of course, I'd had the unusual vaginal bleeding that brought me to the doctor in the first place. Still, I don't think a missed period at forty-eight years of age is something to panic about. I mean, my period returned the next month, only to be followed by another in two weeks. That's when I called the doctor. Let's get real here; missed periods aren't unusual for a woman of any age.

What about the other symptoms? Perhaps if I'd put them all together, I might have been diagnosed earlier.

I studied the photos of our Hawaiian vacation. We'd taken that vacation only two months before all this started. I looked pretty darned good in that bathing suit. No, it wasn't the skimpy bikini of my youth, but it was one that showed off my belly button. It didn't look like I was bloated. Granted, I didn't have the drum-tight tummy of adolescence, but I sure didn't look bloated. So maybe I didn't have an increase in abdominal size.

What about the other symptoms? Looking back, I realized I did have some symptoms. I'd had some constipation, but that happened at the same time as my crazy periods. I took each symptom one at a time and tried to recall the past. I remembered some occasional pain during intercourse. Obviously, it wasn't enough to cause concern. It's not like I suffered when we had sex. I wish I'd been more attentive overall.

Oh yeah, I had one other symptom, shortness of breath. The interesting thing about this is that I was being treated for exercise-induced asthma. I'd had it for years. I used an inhaler prior to exercise and I carried it with me at all times in case of an emergency. Prior to my diagnosis, I'd needed to use it more often than just for exercise. I'd never really thought about it as having anything to do with ovarian cancer, though. I'd had this type of asthma for years before ovarian cancer came into the picture. It wasn't until I was in the hospital that my surgeon even noticed I had an inhaler. He told me I wouldn't need it anymore. I thought, "He must be kidding. I've used inhalers for years. Why wouldn't I need it now? Maybe he means I won't be exercising for a while." But you know what? I haven't had to use an inhaler since. The funny thing is, I do plenty of aerobic exercise such as jogging, playing tennis and riding the stationary bicycle. I am still amazed that I no longer need an inhaler.

Years later, I asked Dr. Friedman about it. I was curious and wondered how he'd known I wouldn't need the inhaler anymore. I was curious to know if my asthma was a symptom of ovarian cancer that I'd overlooked or ignored for years. It gave me the creeps to think that I'd used an inhaler for so long and all along, it may have been related to ovarian cancer. I wondered just how long ovarian cancer had been growing inside me. Could it really be possible that it was there for years and I'd never noticed it?

Dr. Friedman's response was, "Well, I wish I could take credit for curing your asthma, but as far as I can tell there's probably no relationship. I don't think it accounts for things that happen for years before your surgery. I think that in terms of what happened in the months before your surgery, the restriction on your breathing, etc., that would be explained by ovarian cancer, but not things that predated it by years."

Dr. Friedman said that if he'd known that I had exercise-induced asthma, he wouldn't have said anything about my inhaler. He explained that since my abdominal area was distended because of the tumor, he expected that my sensation of shortness of breath would resolve after surgery.

Well, that really left me wondering. If the ovarian cancer didn't cause my asthma, why was I cured of it after my first surgery? Was it simply the power of Dr. Friedman's suggestion that I'd no longer need the inhaler? Perhaps the power of suggestion has more impact than I ever dreamed possible. I just don't know. Maybe the chemo killed my asthma. After all, I certainly didn't exercise during chemotherapy. Is there any chance that it was related to the cancer, even though my doctor doesn't think so? I guess it's just one of those mysteries for which there isn't an answer at this time. All I know is that I don't use an inhaler anymore. All these unanswered questions leave me a little frustrated.

What really upsets me is how uninformed I was about ovarian cancer. Obviously, there are symptoms, no matter how vague they may be. I was angered by the fact that I had absolutely no knowledge of these symptoms prior to my diagnosis. Why in the world isn't this discussed during regular visits to the gynecologist? Why is it only discussed once a woman has the disease?

The sad truth is that only fifteen percent of women are aware of the symptoms. Believe it or not, eighty-two percent of women have never even discussed ovarian cancer with their doctors. I'm no different from most other women who think that getting a good result on a Pap test means there's no gynecologic cancer. I was angry and I wanted to know how to find out if you have ovarian cancer. Surely, there had to be a screening test.

Screening

After my ultrasound detected a large mass, my gynecologist had me come in immediately for a blood test. Surely, *this* must be the way they detect ovarian cancer. The blood test I had was called a CA-125 test. This blood test measures the amount of CA-125, a protein that's increased in the blood of many women with ovarian cancer. Unfortunately, this blood test is not reliable. Some non-cancerous diseases of the ovaries can also increase CA-125 levels. Many women have a

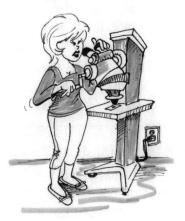

normal CA-125 test result, but still have ovarian cancer. My friend Bonnie had stage IV (the most advanced stage) ovarian cancer, yet her CA-125 test was in the normal range. For these reasons, ultrasound and CA-125 blood tests are not considered accurate enough for screening for ovarian cancer.

At this time, there are no blood tests or imaging studies recommended for early detection of ovarian cancer. The yearly Pap test does *not* detect ovarian cancer; it only detects cervical cancer. My Pap test came back normal, even though I had stage IIIC ovarian cancer. Ultrasound can be helpful in finding if a patient has a mass in her ovaries, but ultrasound does not predict which masses are cancers and which are benign diseases of the ovary.

I guess I am one of the fortunate ones. In my case, the CA-125 test worked. However, at this point, my cancer was already in the advanced stages, so a lot of good it did me! My CA-125 was more than 1,100. It is supposed to be no higher than 35. With no early detection tests available and non-specific symptoms, ovarian cancer has been appropriately labeled "The Silent Killer."

If you have ovarian cancer or if you know someone who does, you will certainly have a lot of questions about the disease. I know I did. At this point, I wanted facts and statistics about this disease. What exactly was I up against? How did I get this disease? How many other women have this disease? Is it curable? I don't recommend dwelling on your disease, but if you are going to win this match, it's important that you understand your opponent. The more educated women become about ovarian cancer, the better chance we have of detecting it early.

As far as ovarian cancer goes, the current recommendation is to do a transvaginal ultrasound every six months with a CA-125 test every three months. While the CA-125 test certainly has a lot of drawbacks, there really isn't an alternative yet. I understand that there are clinical studies and investigations going on right now for an early detection test. I heard this back in 2000 when I was first diagnosed and still nothing has come out. In eight years, you'd think they would have been able to come up with something. The truth is, ovarian cancer isn't common enough to justify routine screening. It's not cost effective. It doesn't matter that it is the deadliest of all the gynecologic cancers combined.

When women see the statistics on ovarian cancer, they are stunned. Simply discussing the statistics with women during their regular exams would surely have many more of them paying closer attention to their bodies. Since there is no early detection test, I think even a pamphlet and a short discussion could go a long way in increasing earlier detection. Apparently, the National Ovarian Cancer Coalition feels the same way. They launched a national campaign called "Break the Silence" in an effort to increase awareness and ultimately improve survival rates.

For me, all this information came after the fact, after the cancer. Even today, as I look at the statistics, I am reminded of my own continuing battle. Yes, the wounds do heal over time, but the scars always remain. And not just the physical scars, either. I have to remind myself that all this knowledge is good. It's knowledge almost every woman with ovarian cancer wants and deserves to know. It just doesn't get any easier to look at. I believe it's important to know your enemy; it truly improves your chances of victory. So, if you need to know the statistics like I did, read on. Remember, they're just numbers, so don't dwell on them. You and I are not numbers!

Statistics

There are lots of statistics out there regarding ovarian cancer and they vary a little depending on the source. The statistics I'm providing are the most common ones I found in books and on the Internet. Keep in mind that statistics change.

- What I learned over the years is that ovarian cancer is the fifth leading cause of cancer death among U.S. women and is the most lethal of all gynecologic cancers. Ovarian cancer kills more women than all other gynecologic cancers combined.

- About 1 in 65 women in the U.S. will develop ovarian cancer and 25,500 new cases are diagnosed each year.

- 14,500 women die from ovarian cancer each year. That's one woman every 35 minutes!

- All women are at risk.

- If ovarian cancer is caught in the early stages, chances of survival are around 90 percent. Unfortunately, only 24 percent of cases are diagnosed in the early stages.

- Around 75 percent of women with ovarian cancer are already in the advanced stages of the disease when they are diagnosed. Of these women, 50 percent will be dead within five years, many much sooner than five years.

- While African-American women may have lower disease rates, their death rates from ovarian cancer are much higher. Only 48 percent survive five years or more.

- My specific concern with survival rates was for patients with Stage IIIC (the stage of my own cancer) ovarian cancer. The estimated five-year survival rate drops below 25 percent when ovarian cancer is diagnosed in Stages III and IV and the overall median survival is 25 to 30 months.

- Many women will be declared in remission or cancer free after surgery and chemotherapy, but recurrence is almost inevitable. Advanced ovarian cancer is now treated as a chronic disease. In other words, you may experience a series of treatments, remissions and recurrences over an extended period.

After seeing those statistics, I was determined to find a way to be in the 15 to 20 percent who would survive five years. I have now survived eight years!

Staging Ovarian Cancer

Staging is a process used to determine the extent of the cancer. Staging ovarian cancer is done surgically. It also enables the surgeon to see if the cancer is confined to the ovary or if other parts of the body are affected. Accurate staging is important because it provides crucial information needed to determine a likely prognosis and to make recommendations regarding appropriate treatment.

There are four stages of ovarian cancer. The first three stages are subdivided into three categories: A, B, C. In very simple terms, "C" is more advanced than "B," which is more advanced than "A."

Stage IV has no categories because it is the most advanced stage. In this book, I will only describe basic staging. I prefer to leave the subdivided categories to the experts as they are beyond my medical understanding.

Stage I: Here, the cancer is confined to the ovary. Phew! This one has been caught early and, not surprisingly, has the best outlook.

Stage II: Here, the cancer has spread from the ovary, but it has not spread very far and is still within the pelvic area. It's getting serious, but it has been caught reasonably early.

Stage III: With this, the cancer has spread far from the ovary and has probably found its way into the lymph nodes and up into the abdominal lining outside the pelvic cavity. Around eighty percent of ovarian cancer patients are diagnosed at this stage.

Stage IV: Now the cancer has spread considerably and has probably found its way into the lungs, liver or lymph nodes in the neck. As with Stage III, cancers at this stage will mean a lot of hard work as treatment progresses.

Gynecologic Oncologists

Most women diagnosed with ovarian cancer end up in the hands of a gynecologic oncologist. At first, this may seem a little frightening. Often women have trusted long-term relationships with their regular gynecologists and don't want anyone else to operate on them. At one time, it was standard for general surgeons and gynecologists to perform ovarian cancer surgeries together, but those days are over. There is a good reason for that, too.

A gynecologic oncologist is a surgeon who deals specifically with cancers of the female reproductive system and also manages the chemotherapy. A gynecologic oncologist is the only physician specifically trained and experienced enough to deal with this deadly disease. A regular gynecologist may see this type of cancer only three times a year, whereas a gynecologic oncologist may see it three times a week or more. The same is true when it comes to an oncologist. An oncologist is unlikely to have the depth of experience necessary for treating ovarian cancer. In these days of medical specialization, it would be difficult to justify any doctor other than a gynecologic oncologist operating on an ovarian cancer patient. Study after study shows survival is markedly improved when a gynecologic oncologist performs surgery. If you appear to have any of the symptoms, or if there is any reason to think you may be at risk, get to a gynecologic oncologist quickly. This should be relatively easy if you live in or near a large metropolitan area. Even if you live in a location where access to a gynecologic oncologist is difficult, you need to find a way to get to one. It really is *that important.*

Remember, seventy-five to eighty percent of ovarian cancer patients don't receive a diagnosis until their disease is advanced. Many of these women have already gone to a doctor with symptoms, but were misdiagnosed because of the vagueness of the symptoms. You can be sure that a gynecologic oncologist is not going to think you are neurotic or being a hypochondriac. Believe me, gynecologic oncologists would rather see patients trust their instincts and seek their help before the disease has a chance to progress.

Rectal Exam

While I'm on the topic of gynecologic oncologists, I thought it might be valuable to bring up this subject. I couldn't help noticing that once I became a patient of a gynecologic oncologist, my pelvic exams included the dreaded rectal exam. I asked Dr. Friedman, "What's up with that? Is this something that should have been included in my yearly routine of the Pap test and pelvic exam? It sure wasn't any part of my exams before."

He chuckled a little, knowing how I felt about the rectal exam. Well come on; it's how everybody feels about a rectal exam! He replied, "In my own opinion, certainly everybody over age thirty-five should have a rectal exam as part of their pelvic exam. Everybody with a posterior tilted uterus should have a rectal exam as part of their pelvic exam at any age because otherwise you really can't assess them very well. And anyone with symptoms should have a rectal exam as part of their pelvic exam.

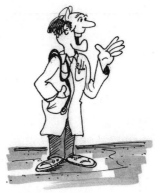

"Now, what can you find? The ovaries tend to be behind the uterus. So the reality is that you're more likely to feel smaller ovarian abnormalities if you do a rectal exam than if you don't. In patients with ovarian cancer, there can be bumpiness in front of the rectum." He said this is called cul-de-sac nodularity.

What he said next surprised me. "I can't tell you how many times I'll do a recto-vaginal exam on a new patient and it will be obvious to me that she has ovarian cancer and nobody ever noticed it before." I asked Dr. Friedman, "You can tell just by a rectal exam?" His reply was, "Just by that!"

I was a bit stunned to hear that a simple rectal exam can tell so much. Not only that, but Dr. Friedman said the same was true for endometriosis. Again, his explanation was, "I can't tell you how many times I've had women come in here and I've felt obvious endometriosis in the area between the rectum and the vagina. I tell the patient then and there without even having to do an ultrasound, 'You know, you have really bad endometriosis.' They ask me, 'How come no one else ever found that on me before?' Well, they never allowed themselves to." As the conversation continued, I listened intently. I found myself wondering; if I had requested a rectal exam, would my gynecologist have even recognized any irregularities?

Okay. So now the lines were getting a little fuzzy for me. I asked, "Is it enough to just get a rectal exam, or does it have to be done by someone who knows what to look for?" His response was, "Yeah, but how are you going to know what you're looking for unless you do them all the time?"

I'm not sure Dr. Friedman's response made me feel any better. He explained that if doctors do more of them, they would get more skilled at figuring out when something is wrong. Another important point he made was that when a doctor does a rectal exam on anyone even close to an appropriate age, it includes a check for occult blood in the stool. That is a screening test for colon cancer. The only bad part of the rectal exam is that people don't like it. It seems to me the benefits far outweigh the brief discomfort of the exam. Ladies, if it's any comfort, this is one test that doesn't discriminate. Men need to get their rectal exams, too. In my opinion, anything that helps in early detection of any type of cancer is a good thing, whether you are at risk or not.

Risk Factors

A risk factor is anything that increases your chances of getting a disease. I wanted to know if I was at risk or even if I had somehow put myself at risk unknowingly. I learned that most women with ovarian cancer do not have any risk factors. Even if you do have some of these risk factors, it doesn't mean you will get the disease. It only means the odds for getting it are greater.

AGE

Age is a significant risk factor. Most women get the disease after menopause. Don't be misled though, because I've met several women in their thirties with the disease. Also, I have read personal stories of women in their twenties who are battling ovarian cancer. Since I hadn't reached menopause, my age did not put me at risk.

OBESITY

I could rule this one out, too, since I've never had a serious weight problem. Many of the women I've met with ovarian cancer were not overweight, either. I found it interesting that this was one of the risks. The American Cancer Society did a study on obesity and ovarian cancer. They found a higher rate of death from ovarian cancer in obese women. The risk increased by fifty percent in the heaviest women.

TALCUM POWDER

Believe it or not, exposure to talcum powder in the genital area may slightly increase the risk of ovarian cancer. Talc in its natural form may contain asbestos, a known carcinogen. Since 1973, all talc products, such as baby powder and body powders, must not contain asbestos. Even though talcum powder is now asbestos-free, studies suggest that when applied to the genital area, talcum powder may affect the outer layer of the ovaries. While the studies are mixed, most experts agree that women should consider avoiding talc products. I don't know how many women use baby powder on their babies, but I'm sure my mom did. I remember always seeing it in the house.

FERTILITY DRUGS

The connection between fertility drugs and ovarian cancer is mixed. Some studies identified certain fertility drugs as increasing risk, while other studies indicate that infertility itself increases risk, not fertility drugs.

I am one of those women who went through infertility treatments in my late thirties. My husband and I made the crazy decision to try to have a child together, even though we were raising his three children from a previous marriage. I'd had a child when I was a teenager, but had given her up for adoption. While I was going through repeated fertility treatments, my daughter, Laura, located me through a private investigator. Now that's a story all on its own, but not for this book. Now that my Laura was in our life, our mission to have another child ended. I was glad it was over. I was emotionally and physically drained from the drugs, the procedures and the failures.

Even while I was going through the fertility treatments, I wondered how the drugs could cause me to produce sixteen eggs during one ovulation. When I asked whether this could produce early menopause or some other complications, I was assured it wouldn't. Looking back, I really have to wonder. I wasn't the only one in my support group who'd taken fertility drugs and ended up with ovarian cancer. In fact, Alisa brought up the subject of fertility drugs. Up until that time, I'd never even thought about the fertility treatments being related to my ovarian cancer. But Alisa had heard there was a connection between fertility drugs and ovarian cancer. She was young and beautiful. She had gone through the whole infertility routine without success, just like me.

MENSTRUAL PERIODS

Women who go through menopause after age fifty, as well as woman who begin having periods before age twelve, have a higher risk. I had my first period at age eleven. So, I guess I can add this to my personal risk list.

PERSONAL HISTORY

If you've had breast cancer, colon cancer or endometrial cancer, you have an increased risk for ovarian cancer. I met several women who had been triumphant with breast cancer, only to end up with ovarian cancer years down the road. I can only imagine how devastating it must have been for these women.

FAMILY HISTORY

If a first-degree relative has had ovarian, breast, colon or uterine cancer, you are probably very concerned – and rightfully so. Women can inherit risk factors from either parent. When there is a family history of cancer, it may be caused by an inherited mutation of the breast cancer gene BRCA1 or BRCA2. Women who inherit these genes are at higher risk.

There are also gene mutations that lead to inherited colorectal cancer and possibly prostate cancer. These gene mutations may also increase risk of developing ovarian cancer. Genetic testing, along with genetic counseling, can determine your risk. Remember, even if you have inherited these genes, it does not mean you will develop the disease, it simply means you are at higher risk.

There's a lot of information available about cancer and genetics. I have only briefly covered this topic. Since I do not have inherited risk factors, I don't feel very knowledge-able on the topic. However, if you are one of the ladies who have inherited risks, you need to realize what this means to you personally. I'm not trying to scare you, but knowledge is power and there are a number of potential genetic mutations that may increase your risk, including some that are more common in Ashkenazi Jews. These are women of Eastern European Jewish decent. My friend Bonnie fell into this cat-egory. So please, if you are concerned or suspect you may have inherited risks, speak with your doctor about genetic testing. It may save your life.

Treatments

At this time, treatments mainly consist of surgery and chemotherapy. Radiation is typically not used for ovarian cancer treatment here in the United States.

SURGERY

Surgery is done to remove as much of the tumor as possi-ble. Ovarian cancer often spreads throughout the abdominal cavity. It can leave seeds or rice-sized implants of tumor on any abdominal organ. The goal of surgery is to remove all cancer that is evident. This is called debulking. Another goal is to do stag-ing. Staging is important for determining chemotherapy treatments and for predicting possible patient outcomes.

The type of surgery you have will depend on how ad-vanced your ovarian cancer is at the time it is detected. It could be as simple as removing an ovary through minimally invasive laparoscopic surgery or it could be as radical as my surgery was. For most ovarian cancer patients, surgery usually involves removing the ovaries, fallopian tubes, uterus, cervix and any other tumor sites.

When I went into the hospital for surgery, I cried in my husband's arms. Crying is not common for me, so you can imagine how frightened I was at the time. I didn't feel sick and that made it even worse. I was getting ready to go through major surgery and I couldn't even look forward to feeling better after it was over. That first surgery was terrifying. I only started to relax once they started administering the drugs. After anesthesia, everything was a haze.

I woke up with hot soft material wrapped all around my head. It was so comforting. But why was my head wrapped? I think it was done to prevent me from going into shock. I didn't care. It didn't matter because it felt wonderful. And an angel was pushing me somewhere on a rolling bed. She was talking to me, but I kept asking her if she was an angel. I got no reply. In reality, she was probably a nurse, but I saw an angel. I don't remember anything else about being in the recovery room. I barely remember anything from my days in the ICU.

I do recall being completely bedridden. I wasn't allowed any food or water during my time in the ICU. I had some type of morphine drip in my spine and I was hooked up to so much crap I felt like I was a machine myself. The nurses were kind and compassionate. I was so grateful for the way they treated me. They gently bathed and cared for me with the greatest regard for my modesty. They were encouraging and helpful. Mostly, I just slept or looked through the window at the gray sky.

It was raining when I went into the hospital and it continued to rain for days. One day, the sun finally broke through the clouds. I opened my eyes to find rays of sunshine flowing through the window to me. I felt the sun's warmth penetrate my skin. There was something very comforting about that time. I never felt as fragile as I did then. Those sunbeams warmed me right through to my soul. That is the clearest memory I have of being in the ICU. I felt I had been touched by something far grander than rays of sun. It was a very physical, yet spiritual, experience. To this day, I feel love and gratitude for those moments.

I had visitors in the ICU, although I can't tell you who came to see me. I know I didn't want visitors. I looked terrible. I don't know why my eyes were swollen or why my face had such a balloon-like appearance. I was pretty miserable, but I guess people needed to see me. I really don't remember much at all about being in the ICU.

After several days, I was moved to a regular room on the cancer floor. Now that's a depressing place. The doctor wanted me to start walking as soon as possible. This wasn't as simple as it sounds. I had been closed with metal staples from my pubic bone to breastbone. There was the catheter to tote. I had two drainage tubes on each side of my pelvis with hollow balls to collect the fluid. The weight of the tubes caused a lot of pain if I allowed them to dangle freely, so I used safety pins to attach them to my hospital gown when I walked. I had two racks of IVs. I still wasn't allowed to have any real food or water, even though I was no longer in the ICU. It took the nurses at least twenty minutes to disconnect and mobilize these things for me to walk. Because it was such an ordeal to get ready for a walk, I made good use of the time. I walked and walked. I visited other patients, I visited the nurses' station and I walked with anyone who would walk with me. The walks made me stronger.

On my last day in the hospital, I finally got some real food, but I hardly ate. Hospital food is pretty gross. At least I wasn't being fed through an IV anymore! I was eager to get home. I was tired of being in the hospital. The doctor showed up early to remove my staples and give me last-minute instructions. Believe me, I was ready to leave, but there was a delay while I waited for a special nurse who showed me how to take care of the colostomy. Luckily, they also provide this care at home for a few weeks until you feel confident enough to handle it on your own. Then finally, I was out of the hospital and on my way home. Unfortunately, I still had the catheter bag that I'd now coined my new purse.

CHEMOTHERAPY

I have so many disturbing memories of chemo that I found myself procrastinating miserably on writing about it. Every time I attempted to approach this topic, I somehow found other things to do. At first, I made sure they were important things that kept me from my writing, but eventually those ran out so even meaningless tasks became a priority. Now that all my excuses have run their course, my only option is to get over it and tell my story as it relates to chemotherapy.

Chemotherapy comes quickly following surgery in order to kill remaining tumors and microscopic cancer cells. My chemotherapy was Taxol and Carboplatin. I received it intravenously, from 9:00 a.m. to 4:00 p.m., every three weeks. It's not just the time sitting with the IV that's maddening; it's also the extensive and specific drug routine that goes with it. I had to take certain pills before, during and after chemo – all in varying doses. It was complicated to the point that I had to post the drug chart on my refrigerator and check off each dose as I took it. They also want you to drink large amounts of fluids after chemo.

The day after my first chemo treatment, I thought, "This isn't so bad. Once I get used to this, it will get easier." Ha! Think again, woman! It wasn't until a day or two later that chemo really hit me. I couldn't get out of bed for one full week without feeling like I was going to pass out. I felt like I had an extreme case of the flu. Every bone and muscle in my body ached. The fatigue was beyond anything I had imagined. It developed into a regular pattern. Always a day or two after chemo, the debilitating after-effects hit. The most discouraging part was that it didn't get better. It got worse. I hoped I was imagining it, but my doctor explained that you don't get used to chemotherapy. It's cumulative. Each treatment gets more difficult.

I wondered how much worse it could possibly get. I knew I had to suck it up and stay strong, but it wasn't easy. The chemo took its toll quickly. My hair started falling out in a matter of weeks. I woke up in the morning with clumps

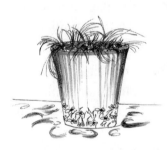

of hair on my pillow. When I brushed my hair, it fell out by the handful. Since my hair was long, there was a lot of it to deal with. Every morning, I filled the bathroom trash can with my hair. It looked like a furry animal lived in there.

What I didn't realize was that my sweet husband frantically emptied it as fast as I filled it. He was afraid I would be too distraught by the sight of it. About a week later, the plumbing backed up and we called Tracy, our plumber, to remedy the situation. Boy was I surprised to hear the plumbing was clogged with hair!

Apparently, Les had been flushing it down the toilet!

Well, we got a good laugh out of that and my husband learned a lesson about what goes down the toilet! And I decided it was time for me to get some wigs.

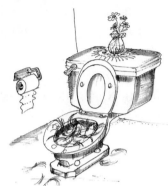

Just weeks after my first chemo, I was bald – and I mean shiny bald! I purchased wigs, hats and sleep caps. While these items can be expensive, most vendors give a discount to chemo patients. Some ladies don't mind being bald, but I wasn't one of them. I felt better with hair on my head. At night, I wore a soft little cap to sleep in. That sexy bald look the celebrities wear just doesn't look the same when you don't have eyelashes and eyebrows. I thought I looked kind of like a Golem or maybe some type of lizard or reptile. I tried to pencil in some eyebrows, but that only resulted in a fit of hysterical laughter. I went from Golem to clown. So I decided I didn't need eyebrows. The bangs on my wig were just long enough to disguise my missing brows.

There are some advantages to being hairless. I no longer had to shave my underarms or legs. Bikini waxes were no longer necessary, not that I'd ever had one. When they say you'll loose your hair, they mean it – every bit of it is gone! At least it's only temporary. It does come back. Be prepared, though, because when your hair comes back, it's different. My mousy brown, flat, straight-as-a-stick hair grew in thick, black and curly. It didn't just happen to me. My friend Bonnie had the same thing. We both looked like Betty Boop! It was cute and fun. Too bad it goes back to its original state after a year or two. To this day, I still don't have underarm hair. My pubic hair and leg hair is there, but much sparser now. Hair loss is the easy part of chemotherapy.

After my first chemo treatment, I developed sores in my mouth. Talk about gross. They were disgusting! I referred to a book the oncologist had given me, *Chemotherapy and You*, by the National Institute of Health. Sure enough, these sores were listed as a common side effect. In fact, all of my side effects were described in simple layman's terms in this informative booklet. Another trip to the doctor for even more drugs cleared this condition quickly.

Food was the biggest challenge. I got so hungry and food smelled wonderful, but even one bite sometimes made me start crying. Everything, even water tasted like metal or dirt. I knew how important it was for me to eat in order to keep my blood count up for the next treatment, but eating became such a challenge. My oncologist gave me a diet most people can only dream of: Eat anything you can, any time of the day – even if it's ice cream for breakfast. Too bad I couldn't take advantage of it. It was especially hard to drink the required amounts of fluid during the five days following chemo. I had to drink eight to ten glasses of any liquid except water (water has no nutrients). It didn't matter anyway, since it all tasted like metal. I managed to force it down with the aid of some incredible anti-nausea drugs. I found that food was easier to get down if it didn't require much chewing. Chewing seemed to bring out the dirt/metal taste more dramatically.

Chemotherapy has lots of side effects. The disgusting taste of food and the nausea were only the beginning. I also experienced neuropathy. Numbness and tingling in my hands and feet drove me crazy. It felt like my feet were asleep. Try to walk when your feet are asleep! I despised walking and the tingling in my hands traveled up to my elbows. Some mornings I could barely open my hands. I hobbled down the stairs and headed straight for the hot tub. This became my morning ritual in order to get my body flexible enough to move. I could no longer wear any of my cute shoes. My feet hurt constantly. I bought tennis shoes in a larger size just so I could tolerate walking.

This side effect (neuropathy) is the result of nerve damage caused by the Carboplatin in the chemo. Once chemotherapy ends, it takes about year for the nerves to repair themselves. In a number of cases, the nerve damage ends up being permanent. Thirteen months after my last chemo, quite a bit of the tingling had gone away, but not all of it. I still had substantial pain in my joints and muscles. I hobbled around stiffly for an hour or so in the morning and when I sat for any amount of time, I'd stiffen up. The only thing that seemed to help was sitting in the hot tub first thing in the morning for about thirty minutes. After putting up with these symptoms for more than a year, I saw a neurologist. The neurologist told me that the nerve damage in my hands and feet would be permanent. Let me tell you, I was not happy hearing that news. I was determined to do something about it. Permanent or not, I was not going to live like this.

Since that time, I've done many things to improve my health and to change the course of my life. I no longer have neuropathy or any abnormal stiffness in my muscles and joints. So, please do not be discouraged by any diagnosis, even when the damage is labeled "permanent" or disease is labeled "incurable." These are just words.

The world is all about change. All things can and do change in our universe. I'm living proof of that. Neuropathy was just one more obstacle to overcome in my stand against cancer. Any way you look at it, chemotherapy is nasty and it comes with a whole bunch of challenges.

For me, the worst part of chemotherapy was the effect it had on my insides. My body felt like there were sinister things crawling inside me. I wanted to shake them out, claw them out or even puke them out. I wanted to scream. I felt crazed at times. Sometimes when I was alone, I would simply lie on the floor and cry, wishing for anything to make it go away. I begged people not to call me during the week after chemo because I was like a train wreck. This was unbelievable to me because I'd always been such a strong and healthy person. Before cancer, I'd participated in all sorts of athletics – everything from off-road motorcycle racing to backpacking to tennis. My endurance and my tolerance for pain had always been extremely high. Now I'd been reduced to little more than a basket case.

All I could do was prop myself up. Looking back, I think I propped myself up pretty darned well. I never let anyone see me during those times. No matter how battered I felt, I made sure I looked good by the time my husband returned from the office. I "put on a face," a wig and got myself dressed, even if it was only an hour before he got home. Any time I was able, I tried to look my best. The week after chemo was hopeless, though. I didn't even try. By the second week, I could pull myself together. It was never an easy week, but I always felt better when I caught my reflection and saw how nice I looked.

I never wanted to look like a cancer victim. That was important in many ways. It always helped my mental outlook. It also helped me feel more positive about my healing. By the third week, I actually started to feel somewhat alive again. I could take short trips to the market or visit with my family or friends. I even attended a few summer parties. The positive feedback I received went a long way in aiding my recovery.

By staying as active as possible while on chemo, I functioned better all around. Staying active also allowed me to meet other survivors by attending a support group at The Wellness Community.

Everyone responds differently to chemotherapy. And not all chemo treatments have the same side effects. Taxol and Carboplatin are really rough. I had side effects others didn't have. Then again, I didn't have some of the side effects others struggled with. Chemo is just horrible, no matter what chemicals are used. There's no doubt in my mind that one day we will look back at this type of treatment in horror. For now, it's the best we have, so we must accept it and move on. I wish I had something more encouraging to say about chemo, especially for those who must face it. Chemotherapy was a nightmare for me, and I'd do just about anything to avoid it. But there was no escape.

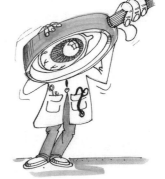

Second-Look Surgery

Many women are extremely frightened to hear that second-look surgery is protocol for ovarian cancer. It's difficult enough to go through the first surgery. Getting sliced open from pubic bone to breastbone is no simple matter. Once chemotherapy is complete (approximately six months for most women), the doctor usually schedules second-look surgery. I've met women who opted out of the second-look surgery, but not many.

Women opt out of a second-look surgery based on a number of weak arguments. Some feel that if their cancer was still present, it would have shown up in the blood tests or in the CT or PET scans they had. After all, if they'd had optimal debulking during their initial surgery and optimal chemotherapy, why go through a second-look? Well, the reality is that these tests aren't accurate indicators. So while these women may have no evidence of cancer after having these tests, about sixty percent of them have a return of cancer. And if cancer is large enough to show up on a CT or PET scan, it would be catastrophic. It would mean that the cancer grew through chemotherapy and that would be a terrible outcome. It has been proven time and time again that second-look surgery is the most effective strategy in determining the status of a woman's ovarian cancer after chemotherapy.

The purpose of the second-look is to see if the surgeon can find any remaining cancer. What your doctor looks for in the second-look surgery is very different from the initial surgery. Your doctor will look for something say, the size of a grain of sand or even smaller – something that can only be seen through a microscope. Dr. Friedman told me he does second-look surgeries with his fingers as much as with his eyes. He *feels* for irregularities as much as he looks for them. The surgeon takes samples and sends them for biopsy. If cancer is found at this time, the doctor has a chance to decide how to proceed. Women with microscopically positive disease often do well with continued chemotherapy.

The type of chemo may change after positive second-look surgery results. It also gives the doctor a chance to switch the patient over to intraperitoneal chemotherapy. Intraperitoneal therapy delivers the medication directly into the abdominal cavity through a tube or catheter inserted into the abdomen.

Any way you look at it, second-look surgery is usually standard for ovarian cancer patients. The decision to have a second-look was one I never had to worry about. I had a colostomy to reverse and because of that, I looked forward to my second-look. And after my second-look surgery, I was declared cancer free!

It doesn't matter whether you are diagnosed with ovarian cancer in Stage I or Stage IV; you will be treated aggressively. That means surgery and chemotherapy. Since second-look surgery remains controversial, you might feel unsure about going through it. It might be helpful to remember that nothing is more effective in discovering the status of your ovarian cancer than the second-look surgery.

You and your doctors are a team now, so you don't need to make these decisions alone. But the choice is ultimately yours. Remember, nothing is etched in stone here; make the decisions that are right for you.

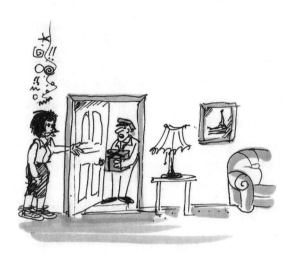

Recurrent Ovarian Cancer

If you have recurring ovarian cancer as I do, please do not give up. I know how bleak the future seems when cancer returns, but your life is important. It may not be your time to leave. When I was diagnosed with recurrent ovarian cancer, I remember thinking I was destined to die quickly. But I was wrong. I'm still here many years later. Consider these remaining years as the most important of your life. Now is the time to choose to be as healthy as you can be in order to fulfill your life in the manner you deserve to live.

Recurrence

It's impossible to discuss ovarian cancer without talking about recurrence. For most women with ovarian cancer, recurrence is inevitable. While statistics always vary, I've read that anywhere from 55 to 90 percent of ovarian cancer patients have a recurrence at some point.

I was completely devastated when I learned of my own recurrence.

Sadly, recurrence leads to a fatal outcome except in the most unusual cases. I know how discouraging this must seem, but remember – I'm still here! That's why I feel my story is important and may prove valuable to others battling this disease.

Dr. Friedman diagnosed my recurrence when he discovered a swollen lymph node in my neck during a routine visit. I was a little frightened when he wanted to biopsy it right there in his office. The thought of him inserting a needle into my neck had me perspiring. But he is so skilled that I felt no discomfort at all. What a relief! Unfortunately, there was no relief when the biopsy results came in. The results were positive. My cancer had returned. I got the bad news when I was in Texas helping my friend Bonnie, who was going through stem cell transplantation at the University of Texas M.D. Anderson Cancer Center.

Bonnie took a different approach than I did when it came to recurrence. Her cancer returned much faster than mine did. She went through chemotherapy again to rid herself of all cancer in order to qualify for the stem cell transplant. Once she qualified, she was off to Texas for many long, hard months of treatment. If the treatment worked, it would mean that Bonnie could look forward to many years free of cancer. It was a risk she was willing to take. With the loving support of her husband, Vince, and several friends, she completed her treatment ordeal. It was a long, hard road, but Bonnie returned home filled with hope.

She often tried to convince me to do the same, but I couldn't do it. It wasn't so much the money as it was the quality of life that influenced me. I just couldn't imagine going through what I'd seen Bonnie endure. I couldn't even handle standard chemo, let alone all the chemo she'd gone through and much more. She was a strong woman, to be sure. I'd rather die than go through what Bonnie did during that stem cell procedure. If my time was limited, I sure didn't want to spend it like that. I give her lots of credit. Believe me, I prayed it would pay off for her. She had so much to live for.

I was so happy when Bonnie came home. We had become great friends. I knew her family and some of her friends. I got to meet her "Little Pineapple," her grandson Conner, who lived in Hawaii. Before Bonnie went to Texas, she and I spent hours creating a baby shower scrapbook for her daughter, Julie. It was filled with pregnancy photos documenting each month from the beginning to the birth of the baby.

I was devastated when Bonnie's remission only lasted a couple of months. We cried and cried. Bonnie's second daughter, Jenny, was getting married and now this. Well, they moved the wedding plans up and decided to have the wedding in Bonnie's beautiful back yard so she could attend. Unfortunately, Bonnie attended the wedding in spirit only. It was a beautiful ceremony and we all felt Bonnie's presence. I miss her so much.

The reason I shared Bonnie's story is to let you know that there are options to explore once you've experienced a recurrence. While this option didn't work for Bonnie, it has worked well for others. I don't really know just how successful stem cell transplantation is for ovarian cancer patients. You'd have to look into it yourself. I suspect the numbers are not very good or we would have heard a lot more about it.

Dr. Friedman said, "What you'll find as you review the recent history of cancer treatments is that some drugs and procedures generate a lot of excitement and then fade away. High-dose chemo with stem cell support is one of those procedures. Our inability to kill every last cancer cell with chemotherapy has often led us to try dose intensification strategies of one sort or another. Bonnie's treatment is a 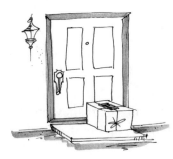 classic example. Every doctor and patient wants to deliver or receive cutting edge therapies. The longer I do this kind of work, the more I believe in the importance of having patients participate in clinical trials."

When ovarian cancer returns, the goal often becomes to stop or slow the spread of cancer, rather than curing it. It is possible that it can be effectively stabilized or treated over an extended period. Many women go in and out of remission. This is why specialists have begun to approach it as a chronic disease. Survivors are not necessarily enthusiastic about this, since it's only "chronic" as long as the treatments are working. The time between remissions tends to get shorter and shorter in duration. The thought of living with ovarian cancer can be overwhelming, but many are doing it and doing it well.

Quality of life should be your top priority. Being well informed will enable you to manage your disease better. By addressing all your needs – social, spiritual, emotional and physical – you can take control of your life. Embrace life, no matter how limited your time may be. As Dr. Friedman says, "This is no time to drink cheap wine."

More Surgery

When it comes to recurrence, the general principle is to start the process again. That means figuring out what part of your body the cancer has returned to and how extensive it is. After the biopsy in my neck came back positive for cancer, I had both a CT scan and a PET scan. Armed with information from these scans, my doctor decided to perform another surgery. This isn't always the case. There is a sort of six-month protocol for both surgery and chemotherapy. If you were cancer-free for less than six months before your recurrence, then surgery isn't an option. The only exception would be if a patient demands surgery or if there's some reason to suspect that the first surgery was not optimal. If you were cancer-free for longer than six months, then the results from scans or other tests may indicate whether surgery is an option for you.

For me, surgery was an option. Cancerous lymph nodes around and under my pancreas, as well as in my neck, were removed during my third surgery. Since I'd had so many problems from the Panacryl suture material, this was also an opportunity to get rid of any remaining Panacryl. In a way, I looked forward to my third surgery and finally ending the Panacryl nightmare. But I soon found out that I wasn't ready at all.

I hadn't realized how traumatized I was from all I'd been through. I started to realize it when they scooted me onto the operating table for the third time. The icy air, the huge circular lamp above me and the routine movements of people prepping the room weighed on me. As they started to strap me down, I broke. I shook and then I sobbed. I couldn't stop the tears. No, I didn't want to do this again! I was scared; and it was something worse than fear. I couldn't control myself. They tried to comfort me with touch and words, but nothing helped. The anesthesiologist came in immediately and, thankfully, that's all I remember.

More Chemotherapy

Even though recurrence may not result in more surgery, it almost always means more chemo. The type of chemo drugs and the way they will be administered depends on several factors. The six-month principle comes into play here, too. If you have been cancer-free for less than six months, it's unlikely that you'll get the same chemo drugs this time around. If your remission was lengthy, you may go back on the chemo drugs that were effective the first time around. If you had some particularly debilitating side effects during your initial chemo, you may receive a different drug.

Even though Dr. Friedman told me I'd definitely have to go through chemo again, I didn't make it easy for him. I'd had such a horrible experience with my initial chemotherapy that I tried everything I could think of to change his mind. Even begging was not beneath me. Prior to my surgery, Dr. Friedman discussed the possibility of trying different chemo drugs with less debilitating side effects. There was a catch, though. He would have my cancer tested for chemo drug resistance. This type of testing is useful in a negative, rather than positive, sense. Dr. Friedman explained that if your cancer grows during chemotherapy testing, then it's very likely that particular chemotherapy drug won't work when it is used in you. The opposite is not true. The chemo may be very effective at killing the tumor in the initial analysis, but it still might not work in you.

So my cancer was tested for chemo drug resistance. Much to my dismay, the three best responses came from Taxol, Carboplatin and Cisplatin. Other drugs weren't even in the ballpark. So I was back where I'd started and would face the same chemo drugs as before. Even though this wasn't what I'd hoped for, it was better than wasting my time on chemo drugs that wouldn't accomplish anything.

The type of chemotherapy you will receive for a recurrence will depend on you and your medical team. Your doctors are key in determining what happens next regarding the type of treatment you will undergo. It's crucial that you have confidence in your doctors. Your faith in them goes a long way towards your recovery and healing. I always knew I was under expert care. I've always had complete faith in Dr. Friedman.

I've found that faith serves me far greater than hope. When I am in a state of hope, I realize I am not here; I'm not living in this moment. To me, hope means something is wrong. Things are bad and not as they should be – and I *hope* things will get better. When I was ill, hope took me away from the moment and put me somewhere in the future. I could hope for a cure, hope to feel better, hope that my kids don't get this one day. I could (and did), hope and hope and hope; but it never changed anything.

Once I started having faith, things got better. Faith grounded me. I had faith that I had the right doctors, faith in their abilities, faith that the outcome would be good. Faith kept me here, where I needed to be. Here and now was where

I savored every moment. Even when I was miserable, I had faith that it would get better. I no longer hope for things. I have faith that things are as they should be. Faith made me stronger. Once I got through that third surgery, I needed faith more than ever, because I truly thought I didn't have much time left.

After surgery, I spent time recuperating and avoiding chemo. I knew I didn't want to go back to the oncologist I'd seen before. I didn't have a specific reason other than instinct. My insistence on change landed me under the care of John L. Barstis, M.D., Medical Director and Clinical Professor of Medicine at the UCLA Cancer Center. Now there's a title! As you know, I was at the point of preferring death over chemo. I needed to let my new oncologist know my feelings. I had no idea how he would respond. His response was to put me on a weekly low dose of Taxol and Carboplatin. Instead of them blasting me with chemo all at once and then having three weeks off, I received chemo in small amounts every week for three weeks, and then I had one week off. This proved highly effective. I didn't know any other recurrent ovarian cancer patients who'd gone through this type of chemotherapy treatment, so I asked Dr. Barstis about it. I was curious about what was behind his decision. Was it because I'd been so adamant about not having chemo or was there some other reason?

Dr. Barstis explained that he'd been involved in a study at UCLA that taught how low doses of chemotherapy could be given weekly instead of one big dose every three weeks. With some of the newer medicines like Taxol, it's just as effective, maybe even slightly more effective, if it's given more frequently because it's always in the body and it works better. If you stay below a certain level, you avoid the amount that makes you so sick. If you can be organized enough to come in every week or most weeks, you can get a little chemo each time. It still adds up to the same amount that you would have received all at once, but it doesn't bother you as much. I couldn't have been more interested. Because of the approach Dr. Barstis took with me, I completed my chemo treatments and led a relatively normal life at the same time.

While this approach worked for me, it may not be the right approach for you. As Dr. Friedman pointed out, not everyone can sit around getting chemo every week. For some, once every three weeks works better. There are advantages and disadvantages to each approach. What's important is to work with your doctor to consider how things will balance out for you. When Dr. Barstis offered that balance, I knew I had found the right oncologist for me.

I wondered if oncologists, like other physicians, specialize in particular types of cancer. Dr. Barstis explained that ovarian cancer is extremely unusual from a doctor's perspective because the surgery is so specialized that it is only performed by a gynecologic oncologist. He said that there are also surgical oncologists, but they only operate on female cancers.

"Unlike almost anything else in cancer medicine, those gynecologic oncologists are also experts in chemotherapy. Most of them don't like to administer chemotherapy, but they do the studies and work with people like us, medical oncologists, to figure out the best chemotherapy," he explained.

Dr. Barstis was well informed about the groups doing these studies and the doctors who belong to the groups and participate in the studies. He told me, "The idea is we do the studies together to figure out the best treatment for ovarian cancer. So the answer is that most medical oncologists don't just specialize in ovarian cancer. We work with people like Dr. Friedman who know a lot about chemotherapy, but don't want to administer it themselves." Your gynecologic oncologist and your medical oncologist will work as a team to determine what type of chemotherapy is best for you.

I was curious about intraperitoneal therapy that administers chemo into the abdominal cavity. I'd heard some hopeful snippets about treating ovarian cancer this way. I asked Dr. Barstis if he did this type of chemo and he replied, "I do. I've done it intermittently through the years, too." He said, "We used to do more than we've done recently." He mentioned a couple of studies that suggest that if this type of chemo is done in the beginning, it can make chemotherapy even more effective.

Dr. Barstis told me, "I think most oncologists have mixed feelings about it because, just like the first time you had chemotherapy, you hated it and it made your life miserable. But next time, we found a way to do it that was effective and it wasn't so bad. Most of the time, intraperitoneal therapy is a pretty nasty thing to go through." Dr. Barstis said that there are situations when he feels it is the right thing to do, but he tries to avoid it. I recalled Dr. Friedman having a similar response, saying that one-third of women weren't able to complete their treatment due to the pain and side effects from intraperitoneal therapy. It is simply too hard on the patient.

Since this type of therapy didn't seem as great as I'd initially heard, I asked Dr. Barstis if there was anything new on the horizon for ovarian cancer patients. He said that ovarian cancer treatment is sort of in a dormant phase right now.

Treatment has gotten better since the invention of Taxol, and it is a definite improvement compared to what was done for ovarian cancer patients ten or fifteen years ago. He said, "A larger number of women do well for a longer period of time. But there hasn't been anything new in the last five years." He talked about how treatments for other cancers, such as breast cancer and colon cancer, have had new developments in something called target therapies that make a big difference. These treatments have not been as effective in ovarian cancer, but the same research is going on for ovarian cancer.

Dr. Barstis is excited about what is going on with UCLA's top doctors in gynecology and oncology conducting basic scientific research. There's a lot of excitement about the fact that if we can understand more about the genetic make-up of cancer cells and how these cells malfunction, it will provide an opportunity to go in and attack those cancer cells. I loved hearing Dr. Barstis say that he has no doubt that we will see some of these new agents come out that will also work for ovarian cancer in the next three to five years.

The reason he feels confident about a new treatment emerging is that ovarian cancer is very treatable. The problem is that ovarian cancer is not curable in a lot of situations. It's chronic, remember? The cancers that have seen the most progress in treatment in recent years are those that are moderately to very treatable with chemotherapy. Dr. Barstis said, "I think ovarian cancer is one where there will be a lot of effective new therapies soon. It looks pretty promising."

When I asked if it was difficult for him to keep up with all the new drugs and treatments, he replied, "It's my passion." That was reassuring to hear. Naturally, keeping up has its challenges and it's impossible to keep up with everything.

But Dr. Barstis thinks most people in his field are passionate about their work. He keeps up by focusing mainly on his area of expertise – oncology and solid tumors. It is encouraging to see the confidence, passion and dedication of Dr. Barstis and others when it comes to treating ovarian cancer. Have faith in your doctors. They are fighting for your life as much as you are.

Because of Dr. Barstis' approach with me, I was able to complete chemotherapy. This time, I had a port implanted in my chest. It looks like a small button underneath my skin and it's hardly noticeable. This port was one of the biggest improvements when it came to my chemotherapy. No more searching and prodding for veins in my arms or hands. I got my chemo through the port. It's a simple and painless procedure. One quick push and the needle is in. There is no pain other than a quick prick.

Even though I haven't had chemo for many years, I still have the port. The best thing about it is that they can use it to draw blood. Since I still need to have blood work done every twelve weeks, the port makes it simple and painless. I don't even give it a second thought. Prior to the port, I dreaded every blood test, every chemo treatment, and that pain of trying to find a vein.

Avoiding stress is crucial to healing. Not only was the port a huge stress reliever, the smaller doses of chemo I received eliminated stress. I didn't experience the devastating side effects I'd suffered through the first time I had chemo. I could drive, eat, drink, think and function as a normal person. I even got my Notary commission during this period. I wouldn't have believed that I would be able study, learn and pass a state exam while on chemotherapy, but I did. I was happy to complete chemotherapy and live a full life at the same time. I am grateful to have landed in the hands of Dr. Barstis. If not for him, I probably wouldn't have gone through chemo a second time and that might have been a poor choice, given the stubbornness of this particular cancer.

Once this final phase of conventional treatment was complete, I went full force into looking for natural and alternative ways to stay healthy. I never wanted to have to go through conventional cancer treatments again. If there was a way to avoid it, I wanted to find it. There is always something new to learn and apply. After chemo, your journey must shift from cancer to regaining your health.

After treatments, you must take back control of your life. It's time to make better choices about how you treat your body. I looked at this time as an opportunity to start with a clean slate. Everything in my body was pretty much dead and gone, the bad along with the good. Now it was time to build it up again.

You get to rebuild your body and bring it back to radiant health. You are starting from scratch, so do it with great care. Nurture yourself. Look at everything and be picky. As you begin, your main focus will be your body. Then your focus will naturally expand to include your mind and spirit. Recreate yourself totally in mind, body and spirit. Do it in the best ways you know possible. You'll find you are an awesome being, an individual with a meaningful life.

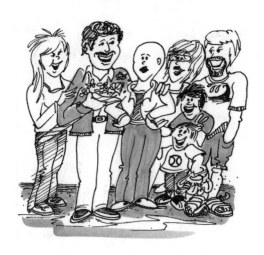

Family and Friends

I don't know about you, but I just hate it when people say, "Oh, you'll be fine. You'll make it. You're strong. You can beat this." I heard comments like those from everyone. And then there's always the standard, "At least they caught it early, right?" Those comments drove me crazy. It made me almost feel like I had to explain or defend myself as to why it wasn't caught earlier.

People think they are encouraging you, but comments like those only leave you feeling worse. While their intentions are sincere, it really downplays the seriousness of your disease. I kept reminding myself that most people are just ignorant when it comes to ovarian cancer and survival rates. Prior to my diagnosis, I was one of those people, too. But when I got sick, I replaced my ignorance with knowledge and I replaced my false beliefs with stark reality.

We all want to believe that our family and friends will rally around us during this devastating time. Obviously, you cannot deal with a life-threatening disease like ovarian cancer without some type of support from family or friends. Your cancer will affect everyone around you in one way or another. Your suffering is inevitable. It isn't easy to see a loved one or a friend going through the torments of cancer. Your suffering will have an impact on them and they will react in unimaginable ways. Relationships will be put to the test during these times.

I was very surprised by the people who were there for me. The people who weren't there for me also surprised me. It's difficult not to have hurt feelings, anger or resentment when someone you expect to support you simply isn't there.

When a neighbor got terribly sick, she was stunned when one of her dearest friends turned her back on her. She quit calling, coming by – she just ended all contact. Now, this was a long-time friend who my neighbor had supported through difficult times and she expected support in return. To top it off, this friend was a medical professional who should have known how important her support would be. My neighbor still carries the pain of this rejection and to this day cannot understand her friend's rejection.

The truth is that some people just can't handle it. Let go of your expectations of others and deal with yourself. There will always be avoiders, people who think that if they hide from the situation, it will go away. For these people, their inability to cope with life's hardships isn't limited to serious illnesses. It is often part of many areas of their lives. Personally, I was not upset by the absence of these people; surprised perhaps, but not upset. I didn't judge them and I didn't hold it against them. I understood completely. I still love them and hold them in the highest regard.

Each person's journey through life has many phases and many lessons. It is not for me to judge another's path. It doesn't matter what the reasons, some people just won't be there to support you through this crisis. Don't focus on who isn't there; focus on who is there and how you can get well with their support and assistance.

Most people don't know how to support you during this time. They don't know if they are helping or getting in the way. The hardest thing for you may be asking for help. I found that when you're able to let people know what type of help you need, most will jump at the chance. It's such a relief for them when they don't have to guess at ways to assist you. I learned that most people provide support within their abilities. Not everyone can be a "nurturing nurse" type. Some people can help by driving you to appointments. Some folks may want to come by just to visit. Some may offer to do the grocery shopping or pick up prescriptions. I was grateful to the many friends, family and extended family members who brought prepared meals to our home. This may seem like a small thing, but to me it was a very big deal. The comfort of home-cooked foods went a long way. Even people who don't normally cook made home-cooked meals and brought them to the house.

Out of this experience, I learned a lot about people and the way they handle or avoid a crisis. I'm fortunate because I have a tightly-knit family. Although each responded differently, for the most part they were there for me with few exceptions. The most vital support came from my husband. While I expected and took for granted that I would receive support from my spouse, I learned this isn't always the case. I've met women whose husbands left them or tried to take away their children because of cancer. I also met women whose husbands mentally abused them or made them feel guilty about the expense or time spent caregiving. I cannot even begin to tell you how much gratitude I have for my husband. He was relentless in his support, even while managing the tremendous workload of tax season. Les is a self-employed accountant, so missing work was not an option for him. How he handled so much stress at one time is beyond me. He never gave up. He was always there for me. He was and remains my hero.

When someone in your family has cancer, it can be all consuming. My husband was completely distraught, yet remained a pillar of strength when he was in my presence. It isn't unusual for the woman to be the foundation when it comes to the family and household duties. Your family lives in great fear during your illness. My sisters told me that it was all they thought about. Whenever they had some down time, there were tears. One of my sisters cried every day on her way home from work. It was particularly hard on my family because I was the big sister who always made things happen. I was the mother who'd always been available for advice, comfort and encouragement. I'd organized the traditional family gatherings.

Just because your children are grown and out of the house, it isn't any easier for them. My children were devastated. They had to nurse their mother, a role reversal that none of them were prepared for, especially considering my history of excellent health. You will find that your illness causes you and your children to worry if this could be something that will be passed on to them. Often children worry if we'll survive to see them marry or have children or if we'll be with them for other major milestones in their lives. So much affects them when their mother's life is on the line. My children still live with memories of how sick I was and how much pain I was in. It was probably harder on them than it was on me. They were all very protective of me.

If your parents are still living, it will be extremely difficult on them, too. My mother definitely went through a lot of heartache throughout my illness. No parent expects to outlive a child. During those first few weeks, after my sister left, my mom stayed with me and cared for me around the clock. Although she kept me in good spirits, she couldn't mask her feelings of helplessness. I could only imagine how she felt. My father had died at forty from a heart attack, so I can't say how a father would go through something like this. I imagine it wouldn't be any easier. The thought of losing a child at any age is terrifying.

Most of my family and friends didn't think I would die. They felt I was a fighter and that I would survive. When my sister Cathy came for visits, she talked about things I had accomplished during my life. She reminded me of how often I had beaten the odds. She told me, "You finished the Barstow to Las Vegas motorcycle race! How many men wish they could accomplish that?" She stressed that I was like a cat, always landing on my feet. She said things like, "Even if the statistics say that only one person will survive, why not you? You can be that one person. I know you can, Chris." I wanted so badly to believe her words, yet I was filled with fear. Everything Cathy said was true. She wasn't simply spouting out "Oh, you'll be fine" platitudes. She sincerely reached out to me and challenged me to pull myself together and use the power she knew was within me. While everyone else seemed to think I would survive, I didn't always have that confidence.

In many ways, my family challenged me, practically daring me back to life. I remember when my sister Carri and her husband Ruben invited Les and me to Las Vegas to celebrate Carri's birthday. That invitation meant a lot to me, since we rarely had the luxury of such time together. I had deeply mixed emotions about it. I really didn't know if I could do it. I was still weak and bald from chemo. My feet and hands hurt terribly because of the chemo-acquired neuropathy and I hobbled around like an old woman. I knew Les wanted to go and everyone was so excited about it. This was going to be another one of life's tests. Saying no would have been the easy way out. I could have used any number of excuses, but I wanted to go, too! It wasn't easy, but I'm sure glad we did it. When I look at photos from that weekend, it reminds me not only of our wonderful time together; it also reminds of my fragile state of mind regarding my own survival.

It's interesting how most of the men in the family were in denial, thinking, "It's not that bad. Lots of people survive cancer." It wasn't until the cancer returned that everyone was forced to face the possibility of my death. These were trying times for all.

Your illness leaves a mark on all those who care about you. It changes your life, and it changes theirs, too. It's important to know it's not all sorrow and sadness, though. In fact, many good things happened because of my illness.

We all became more knowledgeable about cancer. We participated in cancer relays and events, raising money and awareness. We no longer take each other for granted. The best part is our increased focus on living in the moment. I now live a fuller life and so do my family and friends. We relish the joy in life and savor even the simple moments, like when my sister Cathy brought me daffodils in spring, a symbol of hope for a cancer-free world. I consider myself lucky to be surrounded by such wonderful and loving people. It's wonderful to see some of the positive changes that have taken place because of my illness.

I'm fortunate to have a couple of dear close friends. Michele Michaels is one of those rare life-long friends. Although she lives in Washington, she has always found ways to support me. She introduced me to Dr. Hulda Clark's work. Now, because of my issues with cancer, Michele has become quite an advocate for Dr. Clark. Michele made a huge commitment when she started a web site that provides valuable information and products to assist in healing. She tirelessly works this web site, providing monthly newsletters and the latest health information. It warms my soul to realize she did this in an effort to help others – and it all happened because of my illness. You can check out her web site at www.drclarkuniversity.org.

One of the greatest gifts that came out of my illness was a new friendship. Paul and Dolby Dubrow were my husband's longtime friends, but only casual acquaintances to me. So I was surprised when Dolby said she would be at the hospital waiting with my family during the long hours of my surgery. Her support didn't stop there. She brought audiotapes to ease my pain, help me sleep, promote healing and nurture my wounded spirit. There were tapes by Dr. Bernie Segal, Deepak Chopra, Caroline Myss and others. When I was so miserable that I couldn't possibly find anything to feel good about, I'd put my earplugs in, put on a tape and bury my head under the covers until I fell asleep. I always felt better when I awoke. When I couldn't be positive on my own, I let the tapes do it for me. The messages in those tapes truly helped in my recovery. Ever since the day of my first surgery, Dolby has been there for my family and for me. Our friendship has turned into a spiritual journey of soul companions.

When it comes to family and friends, there is much love for you. New doors will open and unexpected gifts will emerge. Even the people who can't support you in person still love you and care about your survival. Stay away from people who are negative, especially if they attempt to lay guilt or stress on you. Stay close to those who have a healing effect on your mind, body and spirit. Most of all, allow yourself to accept help from others. These people want to participate in your healing.

Look for things to be grateful for. It will contribute to your healing. Understanding goes a long way, too. This is especially true when it comes to accepting those who are not able to support you in your healing. Always think loving thoughts about yourself and others. It does no good to harbor negative feelings when your health is at stake. It might be difficult for you, but allow others to help you, even if they are new or unexpected people in your life. These people are in your life for a reason. You need to do everything in your power to enable your healing. Even if you can't see it now, many gifts will come from this experience.

This isn't the time to isolate yourself from the world or from others. The prayers, assistance and love that come from others will have a tremendous impact on your health. Embrace this loving support and always remember to be grateful for everything that comes your way.

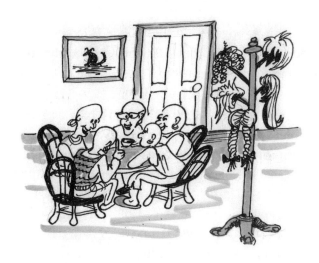

Support Groups

The question of whether a support group will benefit you depends on your personality and the type of support group. Research has shown that cancer patients in general benefit from participating in support groups. However, it is no surprise to me that few patients actually join such groups.

I certainly didn't want to discuss my issues in a group that included men. In fact, I didn't want to discuss my issues with strangers at all! During my chemo treatments, my friend Bonnie asked me to join her in a group at The Wellness Community. My initial reply was, "No thanks, I'm just not into that." Bonnie had attended a few meetings with her husband and it sounded like a pretty depressing group to me. It wasn't long before The Wellness Community formed a group specifically for women with gynecologic cancers. Even though some spouses wanted to participate, men were not allowed to attend. Once the group formed, Bonnie asked if I'd be willing to give it a shot. Since Bonnie and I had developed such a special bond, I decided to be supportive and go with her. I was glad to help Bonnie, even if it meant doing something I really wasn't into doing.

It helped Bonnie because she didn't like to drive at night and she refused to drive on the freeway. Since it was a women-only group, my participation meant her husband wouldn't have to drive her back and forth and then find something to do during the meetings. Believe me; he would have done it in a heartbeat! He would have done anything for Bonnie. I looked at this as a chance to be with my friend and, who knows, I might even get something out of it. As it turned out, I did get something out of participating in that group. In fact, I got more than I ever thought I would.

I met many other women dealing with ovarian cancer. A couple of lucky women had been diagnosed in the early stages, but most were diagnosed in the late stages as I had been. We bonded quickly, exchanged phone numbers and set up carpools. It was a time filled with hope, discussions, learning and exchanging information. My support group was a place where we could talk about things that couldn't be understood by anyone who wasn't in the battle. It was also a place to discuss private issues; things you really didn't want to discuss with others were easy to talk about with ladies having the same struggles. While these were serious issues, we often found ourselves laughing at how we attempted to overcome some of our problems, particularly some of our sexual challenges.

Some problems were unique to specific individuals, such as me with my Panacryl issue. I was the only one who'd had Panacryl suture material, so I got to show my sutures and open wounds to group members. The packing procedure alone was enough to send everyone running to their doctors to confirm that Panacryl hadn't been used on them!

Some of us also had problems with neuropathy from chemo. As a reminder, neuropathy can cause tingling or numbness in your hands and feet. For some ladies, neuropathy was debilitating to the point that it affected their ability to drive and walk. There were all sorts of discussions about how to remedy neuropathy. A supplement called L-glutamine really seemed to improve the condition. I took L-glutamine, an amino acid, faithfully for years. It seemed that all the women in the group did something on their own to contribute to their healing. Just learning about what others did was informative and motivating. It was fun to try new things.

The Wellness Community offers programs on relaxation and guided imagery, yoga, stress management and more. I attended presentations where doctors and other highly qualified professionals shared the latest information. This is a place where anyone involved with cancer can find support. It doesn't matter whether you're a patient, spouse, child or friend – there's a place for you here. If you don't have a Wellness Community in your area, look into other organizations nearby that offer this type of support. You don't have to go through this alone, and neither does your family.

I learned a lot during the time I spent at The Wellness Community. I was most surprised to learn that nearly all cancer patients seek ways to participate in their own healing. These people were no different from me. They tried lots of alternative and complementary therapies. I hadn't heard of many of them until someone in the group brought them up. That gave me new avenues to explore. I realize that support groups aren't appropriate for everyone, but for the most part, I found myself pleasantly surprised by the experience.

As time moved on, the group went through lots of changes. Members came and went. Remissions came and went. About ten of us attended consistently. There were some absences due to medical treatments out of state or out of the country. For me, though, the advantages of participating in a support group eventually waned. It happened very slowly. I think it was a result of dwindling success rates. Our group, once filled with such hope and expectation, was now filled with recurrences and remorse. Funerals marched on in succession as members lost their lives.

The Grim Reaper had a name and it was Ovarian Cancer. I hated it. Our group was literally dying out. I felt like I was in some sort of sick lottery, just waiting for my number to come up. I finally left when Bonnie died. I just couldn't take it. I found that I'd taken on the burden of others' illnesses. These were people I'd cared about and now they were gone. I couldn't bear to look at new members and think how this relentless disease could too soon crush all their hopes. It just wasn't something I wanted to continue.

I was thankful for everything The Wellness Community had given me, but it was time to move on. If I was going to beat this disease, I needed to stop talking about cancer. I needed to stop thinking about cancer. I needed to remove the negative influence of hearing about, and being around, recurrence and death. Most of all, I had to stop "living" cancer. I needed to find a path of joy and strength. I suppose all things must end – or so they say. It was no different for my support group. It had served its purpose and I was grateful for that. I will always be grateful for the wisdom, the friendships and the coping strategies I gained during my time at The Wellness Community. Joining a support group has both advantages and disadvantages. The choice is yours.

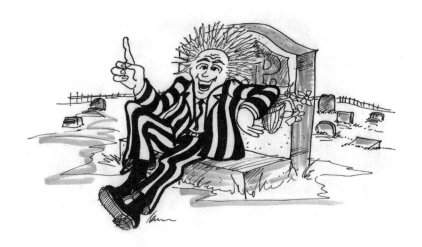

The Plot Thickens

While I counted down what at times seemed like endless days, I couldn't help but wonder if I was prepared for death. I don't mean mentally prepared, but was I prepared on the physical level? I was grateful that my husband and I had set up a Living Trust, but I wanted to review it and make sure everything was in order. I know several people who decided to set up a Living Trust or a Will during this time. Most do so with the emphasis being that it's something they should have done long ago or they are at an age that it needs to be done anyway. This helps because it makes the task more routine than cancer-driven. Healthy or not, it's a comfort to know that your assets will be distributed according to your desires, and not the desires of the state.

If you set up a Living Trust or a Will when you have cancer, it doesn't mean you have given up or that you believe you will soon die. Most women who do this remain hopeful, wanting to complete their treatments and it put it all behind them. It's just that it's practically impossible to get a cancer diagnosis and not think about dying. The word "cancer" alone brings thoughts of death and suffering. Cancer invades your life, disrupts your home and work routines and even your thought patterns. It forces you to think about death in ways you may have avoided. Most of your avoidance is evident by your lack of preparations.

Cancer can motivate you into getting the details of your life in order. The simple act of setting up your Living Trust or a Will can contribute to your healing. It's one less thing to worry about and one less thing to cause stress. It's well known that worry and stress have a negative impact on health. While most of your thoughts are focused on treatments and recovery, it's impossible to avoid thoughts of death and how to prepare for it.

Consider items that may not make it into your Will or Living Trust. Treasured items such as your jewelry box, a special book or something in the curio cabinet might get you thinking. There were some keepsakes that I wanted to go to specific family members, but I wasn't sure about other items. So I decided to ask family members to identify items that had special meaning to them. If there was anything in particular that they'd always admired or wanted, then I wanted to know about it. My children were a bit taken back, wanting to know why they should tell me this now. I tried to make light of it with weak explanations and I even tried to make a joke of it. Without hesitation, they stepped up to the plate, teasing me right back. They joked about how I was going to wake up the next day and see everything tagged with Post-Its. Pink for one child, blue for another...and on they went identifying colors for everyone. They were relentless. Soon we visualized the house plastered with a rainbow of Post-Its. They described Post-Its on everything from the logical to the absurd. They had great fun at my expense and all I could do was laugh along with them.

Eventually, they came to terms with my request and identified those few items that had special meaning to them. I did this with other family members. I added these items to my own list of distributions and put it with the copy of our Living Trust. It's interesting how my perspective on these items changed after that. Just knowing how others felt about these possessions or hearing some special memory attached to an item changed my view of it. I found myself giving many of these gifts away then, rather than waiting until I die. I experienced great joy in doing so.

From the time of my initial diagnosis, I knew there was the possibility of death. I had been closer to death than I wanted to admit; yet its full impact never hit me until two years later when the cancer returned. The five-year count-down ended abruptly. I knew exactly what it meant to have recurrent ovarian cancer. I knew the pattern all too well. It was over. I would die of this disease and chances were it would happen pretty quickly. I knew I wouldn't check out the next day, but the years ahead were numbered. I began to address preparations for my death.

Once again, we reviewed our Living Trust, only this time it involved a trip to our attorney to ensure that additions we'd made were legally in place. I began to think about funeral preparations. I'd never considered where I would be buried. I'd always assumed I'd be cremated. I struggled with these thoughts until I could no longer keep them to myself. I decided to discuss it with my husband. Believe me, it wasn't an easy discussion. First, he didn't want to talk about it. He was having a difficult time coping with the concept of losing his wife. Once he realized I wasn't giving up the fight with cancer, he relaxed and opened up to the discussion.

As I expressed my desires and concerns, Les listened closely. I thought I should be cremated and put to rest in the mausoleum next to my father, who is in a different cemetery than the Bledy family. My rationale was that Les was still young and would most likely remarry. Not only that, but his next marriage could last longer than ours had. What was he going to do, bury one of us on each side of him? I knew she wouldn't want that! While Les appeared to be listening patiently, I sensed his alarm. Even so, I pushed on with other absurd concerns regarding my funeral and the accompanying arrangements. When I finished, Les started. Boy did I get an earful!

To sum it up, I am no longer attached to being cremated. After all, what do I care? I mean really, I will be dead and gone. If it means that much to him and the family to have me in a casket at the funeral, who am I to take that away? Not only that, but Les made a good point. What if he doesn't remarry? No one knows the future. He reminded me that I am a Bledy and this is my family. These are my children and grandchildren. I saw his heartache as he asked, "How could you take that away from me?" He was right. Once I'm dead, it's no longer about me. It's about the family, the living and the grieving. It should be done in a way that serves them best. He was right about all of it and I told him so.

Les was obviously relieved to see that I had come back to my senses. Perhaps it was his relief or maybe he knew it should be done, but either way, he agreed it was time to purchase our cemetery plots. I made an appointment with one of the family services directors at the cemetery. Hearing this, our children and others worried, secretly thinking we weren't telling them everything. By the time our appointment rolled around, we had done a lot of joking and kidding about it. Mostly we did it to ease others' worries. Besides, why not have fun with it? We couldn't change anything.

Our teasing and joking wasn't limited to family and friends. We had a lot of fun making the guy at the cemetery squirm. He couldn't quite tell if we were kidding or serious. After all, Les and I both looked pretty young and healthy. We were smiling and happy as we discussed possible purchases. We knew there was nothing available where most of the family is buried. The few remaining plots had been assigned to family members decades ago. Our generation would rest in a new location up in the hills with a view. We were surprised when we learned the only plots available hadn't yet been developed. It would be a year before they would be ready. We viewed the undeveloped area and selected our plots.

Once we got to the paperwork, Les asked if he could have a refund if I died before our plots were ready. Stammering a bit, the director explained they would put me in another area. Les boldly stated, "My wife has cancer and she could die any day now." Now the director really wondered if this was a joke or if Les was being serious. It was a little hard to believe, given our cheery attitudes throughout the process. Les continued to tease him, saying he thought there wasn't anything else available. That led to more explanations. Les teased on, asking where they would bury him if I ended up in one of the other areas. Would they squeeze him in beside me or would they have to put him on top of me? On and on he went. I laughed the entire time, knowing Les was getting such a kick out of it. Although we came clean with the real story, the director's pleasant smile and thoughtful expression couldn't hide the fact that the truth wasn't much more comforting. The fact was that I really could die before the plot was ready, but we were tired of drama. We looked at it in the same way we look at buying insurance. We have it just in case, because it's typically when you don't have insurance that you need it the most.

Lots of people were uncomfortable when they learned we purchased cemetery plots during this time. Actually, it turned out to be a bonding experience for us. We found comfort and joy in the process. We didn't know how much time we had left together and in a way, it didn't matter. We spent each day living in the moment and finding whatever joy we could at the time. In a way, it was an intimate time that brought us closer. We gained newfound knowledge of each other. Since purchasing our plots, we have visited them to ensure they are complete and to see what the area looked like once finished.

We have also attended funerals there since our purchase. One funeral led us to the same area of our own plots. Our daughters' close childhood friends were twin sisters. When the twins' father died, we all attended the services. Their father is buried in the same section where Les and I have our plots. In fact, you must pass our plots to visit his. It was such a strange feeling that day, seeing the kids comforting their friends, all of them grown up now and most with families of their own. Seeing them together at the gravesite, know- ing that was where they would come to visit our generation.

Knowing the twins would remember us as they passed our graves on the way to visit their own parents' graves and knowing our children would do the same. I wish there were words to describe the feelings I experienced that day. I felt spiritually and peacefully connected with all things. I could see my role in the great cycle of life and death. I could see it because it all took place near my own future gravesite. The whole experience reaffirmed that I'd made the right choice in selecting and purchasing a plot.

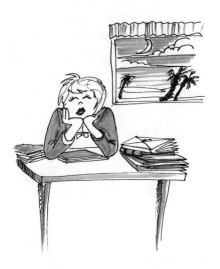

My Stinking Thinking

When you have cancer, you'll find that everyone has an opinion. When I felt well enough to read, I tried to get my hands on anything and everything that had any information about curing cancer. I started with the many books and tapes I'd received from well-meaning family and friends. There is some fascinating information out there – and a lot of it, too! It seemed there were endless books and tapes on the subject, not to mention countless web sites. As a result, I got lots of opinions.

I read medical, spiritual, nutritional and other types of information as it relates to cancer. As I started my research, I realized how often the writers and speakers talked about attitude. Well, I was in for quite a shock when just about everything I read or heard said that I'd made myself sick. Oh yeah, and the one feeling I got out of most of this information was guilt! Yes, I said guilt! I read that cancer is always your fault for one reason or another. I had gotten sick because of the way I thought. My chakras were out of balance, I had bad karma, I wasn't religious enough, I was too active, not active enough and I was eating wrong, sleeping wrong and probably just living wrong. The reasons varied, but it always came back to being my own fault. It got to the point that I didn't know where or how to begin with myself. And all this time I'd thought I was a positive, happy and well-balanced person. Boy, I was screwed!

Apparently my *"stinking thinking"* had made me sick! I sure didn't like that, but I was willing to take a critical look at myself. I'd do anything to stay cancer free. With real honesty, I repeatedly reviewed and evaluated my life, my self-talk patterns, my actions, my treatment of others and my genuine gut feelings. I really had a hard time assessing my thinking.

The problem with this was that I just wasn't a negative person. In fact, I'd always had a keen awareness of the effects of negative self-talk and destructive behaviors. It just didn't add up for me. I am one of those people who jump out of bed early in the morning, cheerful and happy. I am one of those people who find the positive side in every bad situation. I am one of those people who always notice the beauty in my surroundings. It is not unusual for me to thank God for a beautiful day or an awesome sunset. I'm in awe of the stars and nature, but I also enjoy my work and everyday challenges that come with jobs and families. I rarely let things frustrate me or bring me down. So where was my negative thinking?

It got to the point where I actually started to get depressed. Not just depressed, but truly guilt-ridden. According to what I read, somehow I had given myself cancer by the way I thought and lived. Apparently, stinking thinking includes negative self-talk, mean and unkind thinking, even harboring hate for those who have done you wrong. Again, I scrutinized my past and those who'd had any type of negative impact on my life. Once more, I simply was no longer angry with these people and I wasn't hiding any unresolved issues – or so I thought.

Very early in life, I had been fascinated with religion. I'd tried just about all of them and found I was most interested in Buddhism, particularly Tibetan Buddhism. It was here I learned about true forgiveness and how to let go of destructive thoughts. This is done internally and it doesn't come easily. Hanging on to destructive thoughts, not forgiving others and trying to punish others not only wastes time, it also damages us. It can injure us mentally and physically. Learning to forgive is challenging, yet once it's done life gets much better.

Life is one big school. It's all about lessons and learning. Some of my favorite books are by the Dalai Lama and Pema Chödrön, an ordained Buddhist nun, although Lobsang Rampa's books got me hooked on Tibetan Buddhism. I was quite young then. Lobsang Rampa wrote lots of books and I think I read all of them, some more than once. It was through those books that I developed an interest in the Dalai Lama and the ways of Tibetan Buddhism.

I can't imagine how sick I would have been if I had been an outwardly negative thinker or a highly stressed person. That isn't to say I've never been stressed out or made bad decisions. After all, I'm only human and I've had plenty of challenges in life. I've had more than my share of hardship and I've learned many difficult lessons, but I've always been grateful for those experiences. They made me a better person in the end. I have no bitterness, regrets or anger about my life. I simply am who I am.

Now, don't get me wrong, I do take responsibility for my disease. Certainly, something gave me this disease. While my harmful thinking may not show up in the obvious, I figured it had to be lingering in me somewhere. But it would be a daunting and frustrating task for me to go around trying to change every single thing about me when I didn't really know the cause of my disease. The worst part was the guilt I put on myself from everything I learned about how our minds cause sickness. It kind of got me crazy. It seemed to always come back to me. Somehow, I had made myself sick with my stinking thinking.

As I attempted to evaluate and identify my destructive thoughts, I looked at everything I was and wasn't doing at that time. For me it boiled down to an in-depth reality check. If I tried to do all the things suggested, I would surely be a candidate for therapy! Think about it. You'd be trying to meditate, balance your chakras, get Reiki healing, acupuncture, acupressure, find God, go to church, find new doctors, get new treatments, take vitamins, eat herbs, buy supplements and I'm sure the list could go on and on.

The main thing I want to pass on to you from all this is that you need to STOP BLAMING YOURSELF! Accept that, yes, you do have a disease. Things you've done may have caused or assisted in the progress of the disease. However, this is not the time to feel guilty about your disease and what you might have done and it isn't the time to blame everything on your thinking or your lifestyle. Now isn't the time to turn into a big ball of guilt! It will not help in your healing.

Now, with that said, let me make sure you understand that your thinking, whether it is negative or positive, *does* affect your health. There is so much information on this subject when it comes to cancer (or any disease, for that matter) and it surely does have an impact. The way you think is crucial if you are going to be serious about your healing. If you are a negative person or if you have never listened to the way you speak to yourself, now is the time to make some changes. Self-talk is powerful – so powerful that it can change your life.

Start listening to the way you talk to yourself. You'll find that you beat yourself up for the silliest things. You say things to yourself that you'd never say to another person. Take a sensitive situation, for example. Perhaps a friend is upset because she failed at an important task or maybe she made a bad decision. Think about the way you would respond to that friend who comes to you distressed over the matter. What would you say? How would you try to make her feel? Would you tell her that she had done a stupid thing and that she was incompetent or awful for what happened? Would you mentally beat her up with harsh words and criticism? Probably not. You'd probably be quite kind and caring. You would probably say encouraging or loving things. Chances are, you'd be supportive and understanding.

Why would you behave this way with your friend? Think about it for a minute. Now ask yourself; if *you* made this very same mistake or had this exact same failure, what would your self-talk be? Most of us would say terrible things to ourselves. We would be very harsh and critical.

Oftentimes, we call ourselves "stupid" or use other negative words to describe our behavior. Now, why would we treat our friends so kindly and treat ourselves so terribly? It doesn't make sense.

Some of the wisest advice comes from Louise L. Hay, author of *You Can Heal You Life* and many other books. She recommends that you go to the mirror and look directly into your own eyes. As you do, say, "I love you" to yourself. She even recommends that you use your name. Say it aloud and truly and feel it. It takes some practice, but you'll get past that uncomfortable feeling. She feels this practice reaches the inner child in all of us and can stimulate much healing. If haven't read her work, I recommend it. Her personal story and teachings have benefited people all over the world.

So pay attention to your self-talk. Listen closely and any time you speak poorly of yourself or to yourself, STOP! Immediately replace your negative talk with something positive. I'm not saying that you should lie to yourself in order to feel better because lies won't work. Be honest and be truthful, but always be kind to yourself. Speak to yourself in a way that has a positive effect. Say it as if God is listening. Speak as though the words you say are going to be etched on your tombstone. Be to yourself what you would be to others if you knew God was watching you at that very moment. You will feel good when you take this perspective. It is humbling, yet the right words will come.

You don't necessarily have to be a negative person to say negative things to yourself. Even if you are not thinking pessimistic thoughts on the whole, please take time to listen to your self-talk. This is especially important now, because you've been diagnosed with a life-threatening disease. You need to be sure that everything you say to yourself has a positive effect on your healing. Even though I am a positive person on the whole (sometimes accused of wearing rose-colored glasses), I still have to deal with cancer and that means dealing with an enormous range of emotions and thoughts that come along with the disease. Stinking thinking isn't all encompassing. You don't have to be angry and unhappy in order to have damaging thoughts going on in your head.

While you will be able to recognize your self-talk patterns quickly, you also need to look at the not-so-obvious. By that, I mean look below the surface. In order to survive and remain sane, we often suppress many emotions. There may be unresolved feelings of anger, hurt, abandonment or other issues under the surface. It is extremely important that you address these issues and resolve them once and for all. Think about people who have hurt you. Thoroughly visualize or write about these situations in as much detail as possible. Even if the person is dead, you can still talk to them or write to them. Tell the person how the experience made you feel and how it has affected your life. Say or write everything you have in your heart – no matter how ugly it seems. Then tell the person you forgive them. Let that person go. Send them to God with love. If not God, then send them to the light or wherever is good for you. Be sure to send them with love and forgiveness. It will release you. It will lift you. Most of all, it will free you. I believe it frees the other person, too.

Letting go with love and forgiveness may take time, but the payoff is worth it. When you do this, you will notice a lightness of spirit. It releases so much suffering; suffering that you have been carrying around with you all this time and didn't even realize it! Some folks choose to write about these feelings and situations in a journal. Others use visualization techniques. Some actually mail letters or even make phone calls to people who have hurt them. It is not necessary to make actual contact, although many do. It is enough to simply go through the exercise alone. But remember, you must be able to actually forgive and release these people with love. If the situation was so horrific that you just can't do this, then at the very least release the person to God. Turning it over to God or Source will at least free you of the burden.

This technique also works for you as it relates to people *you* may have hurt. It works if you have wronged anyone or have feelings of guilt about any situation. Sometimes people even have guilt about how they treated animals or other circumstances that may not involve people. Use this exercise to resolve those issues once and for all. It's not an easy exercise, but it is most beneficial and will help in all areas of your life. In fact, everyone should do this exercise; even people who aren't ill. It's one of those things that, simply put, elevates your progress as a human and assists in your spiritual development. These issues are surely a part of your destructive thinking that must be resolved if you are ever going to get healthy.

My negative thinking was far deeper than I'd thought. If you are a positive person by nature as I am, then it will take some real soul searching to get to the source of that thinking. It wasn't until I cleaned out the basement of my soul that I discovered there was a dungeon below it. This frightened me, since I thought cleaning the basement was my goal. Suddenly, I had to face the fact that this task had served only one purpose and that was to locate my dungeon. Although I was afraid to descend into this gruesome place, I did it. Like all dungeons, it was filthy, well hidden, soundproof and locked up tight. Here, I found plenty of unhealthy thoughts, along with people I had imprisoned and situations I had locked away. You do not go to a dungeon for a picnic; there is difficult and serious work to be done. Once I'd discovered my dungeon, I couldn't ignore it. I needed resolution in my life and time was running out. I chose to deal with my dungeon, since that's where most of my destructive thinking was hiding and thriving. Just because I had to go to my dungeon, doesn't mean you will have to go to yours.

Monitoring your thoughts and changing your thinking doesn't have to be complicated. Don't feel like you have to go on a spiritual quest or visit your dungeons to improve your thinking. You can make great strides in your healing simply by becoming aware of your thoughts. If they are negative, reform them into something positive and healthy.

The way you think involves the choices you make. If you decide to win the cancer battle, then you have just made a choice. The choice to win means you will have a lot to think about and a lot to do. Any time you make a decision or a choice, you are thinking. Since you think you will win, you must act in ways to accomplish it. Even if you have been told there is no hope for a cure, your thinking and your choices can prove differently! Doctors are not gods. They are human beings just like the rest of us and believe me; they see miracles all the time. Many people have been on death's doorstep with no hope, yet they are alive and healthy today.

The way you think affects the choices you make. Healing is all about those choices. The way you think about your cancer will affect the way you manifest your cure. The process of healing involves your total self. By that, I mean you must heal all parts of you. It isn't just your body that needs healing; it's your mind, your body and your soul. Once you accept this, then you can take actions that will result in complete and true healing.

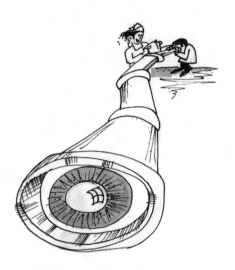

What Is Your Focus?

What exactly are you focusing on? This is perhaps the most important question you can ask yourself. At one time, I truly thought I was focusing on the right things when it came to my disease. I was eating healthy so the cancer wouldn't come back. I was exercising regularly so the cancer wouldn't come back. I was drinking lots of water so the cancer wouldn't come back. I was getting lots of fresh air and spending time outdoors so the cancer wouldn't come back. Everything I was doing, I did so the cancer wouldn't come back. Well, guess what? The cancer came back. You see, my real focus was on the cancer coming back.

I wouldn't have realized the importance of focus if it hadn't been for my friend Dolby. She has always been there for me, through thick and thin. Dolby is one of those special people who consistently grows and learns to achieve balance with mind, body and spirit. When she finds something she believes is valuable, she passes it along to me. My shelves are filled with books, tapes and CDs. Many were given to me and many I found on my own. Dolby introduced me to a wonderful book and an awesome DVD that helped me realize I had been focusing on the wrong things. I'm not saying I was being negative, because I wasn't. I'm usually positive and happy. I just didn't realize the many ways I had been sabotaging myself. It was enlightening and exhilarating to learn how to make this change. It doesn't matter if you are sick or healthy, depressed or happy, lonely or loved, rich or poor, I highly recommend the following:

1. The book, *Ask and It Is Given*, by Esther and Jerry Hicks
2. The DVD, *The Secret*, based on the book by Rhonda Byrne

These two resources are affordable and easily attainable. They have helped more than anything else in my life. Unfortunately, they weren't available during the early years of my cancer misery, but now they are the foundation of my continued health. I am not just speaking about my physical health, but all areas of my life that needed improvement. There is no work or preparation required, only that you have fun. That's the best part, the fun.

It's not about positive thinking, although that is very good. It's really about the things we focus on in life. The most important concept I learned from these sources is that it doesn't matter if I say "No" to something or if I say "Yes" to something, if I am focused on that thing, then it will come to me.

When I was doing things so my cancer wouldn't come back, I was really focusing on my cancer coming back. It was "MY" cancer and I referred to it that way. My cancer, my treatment, my illness, my, my, my… I really owned that disease! When it came back, I was devastated. I couldn't understand how the cancer was back when I had done so many healthy things. You see, it had been all about *my illness* – not *my health.*

When I think back to my cancer support group, it's clear that we were all focused on our illness instead of on our health. My friend Bonnie was so focused on her disease that she had copies of every procedure, surgery, test, drug, chemotherapy and any document related to her ovarian cancer. Her home files were packed with all this information. I remember a time when she asked me why I didn't have copies of this information. She was horrified to know I didn't have this information at my fingertips. What if my cancer returned? Wouldn't I need that information? I think that instinctively I must have known this wasn't a good thing. I told Bonnie, "That's Dr. Friedman's job! If my cancer comes back, it's his job to deal with all that information." She thought I was being careless and expressed her concern. Bonnie and I became great friends through our struggles with ovarian cancer, but we approached our healing differently.

I don't think it helped when they started treating ovarian cancer as a chronic disease. It was bad enough to know the grim survival statistics for ovarian cancer patients, but now we had to face the fact that for most of us, the disease would continue to return until we no longer responded to treatment. That really sucked. As expected, my support group members continued to die off one by one. The focus was no longer on being cured; it was on how long we could survive. Who would be the next to die? Finally, after most of the initial group died, including my precious Bonnie, I dropped out of the group. It was time to change my focus. I did this instinctively, since I did not have the benefit of *The Secret* or *Ask and It Is Given* at that time.

I had to find a way to focus on health, longevity and wellness. I decided to stop talking about my disease, cancer and anything related to my illness. This wasn't easy and anyone with cancer knows how difficult it is. If I started to think about my cancer, I forced myself to stop. The only way to stop a thought is to replace it with something else. I forced myself to say things in my mind, such as, "Thank you for my healing" or "I am so grateful for my improved health." I thanked God for the beautiful day, or for my husband, family or home. I thought of *anything* positive and wonderful that I could create at that very moment. Then I purposely continued to conjure up lots of good thoughts for a long time or as long as it took to really change my thinking.

It takes a conscious effort to monitor your cancer thoughts, but once I started doing it, I became aware of how often I thought about my cancer. It took quite some time before I was able to get through a day without talking about it, let alone thinking about it. As you begin to monitor your thoughts, you'll begin to realize that your self-talk isn't always nice. You'll find that you often use kinder words to speak to strangers than you do to yourself. I'm not saying that you should lie to yourself. Just change your negative or fearful thoughts to thoughts that are healthy and beautiful. Once you start doing this, it becomes easier. In fact, it can be fun. After a while, I found I'd started thinking wonderful thoughts all on my own without even needing to prompt myself. Slowly, my focus was changing.

I stopped looking in the obituaries for cancer victims. I no longer browsed through the bookstore for books or magazines about ovarian cancer. In fact, I have quit exposing myself to lots of negative things. I've even stopped watching the news on television. Now I skim through my morning newspaper, focusing on good news and then briefly check out the rest. I want to stay informed, but I don't need to be inundated with the horrible details, especially on a daily basis. Changing what you focus on can have a tremendous impact on your recovery and cure.

Don't watch violent or depressing movies. Watch as many comedies as possible. Laughter is wonderful for healing. Enjoy reading and watching things that make you feel good about yourself or things that contribute to your health and wellness. I continually look for ways to improve my life in all areas. Don't just limit your focus to improving your health. There are many other things to live for, too. Focus on love and find ways to be grateful. Even if you can only be grateful for small things, do be grateful for them. Your love and appreciation creates wonderful energy. It's so much better than feeling terrible or fearful about things.

I think back to the stories I've read about people who have beaten the odds with cancer. Many of these people, like Lance Armstrong, had no real chance of surviving, yet they did. I was glued to his book; it is one the most inspirational stories I've ever read. Not only did Lance survive, he thrived – winning the Tour de France a record-breaking seven times. I find it interesting that in the survivor stories I've read, all had one thing in common. At some point, they shifted their focus. I remember reading how stunned Lance Armstrong was in hearing that his physician, Craig Nichols, wanted to tailor his treatment to get him back on the bike. Lance just wanted to live, but Dr. Nichols felt that he could race again. The shift in focus went from the possibility of dying to the possibility of competing again. Although this possibility was completely off the radar for Lance, the doctor planted the seed.

These shifts are rarely instantaneous. A shift in focus is nurtured slowly and continually. Shifting your focus from, "I just want to survive" to "Look at me, I'm on top of the world" takes time. It's not going to happen overnight. If you read Lance Armstrong's book, you know that for him, the shift occurred in many phases and it wasn't until he regained his health that he even dared to try to race again. I just know that when I read survivor stories, I notice turning points in their focus.

In my mind, I hear the voice of Esther Hicks explaining how it doesn't matter if you shout, "Yes" at something or if you shout "No" at that same thing, the fact that you are shouting at that thing will manifest it. Well, now I chuckle at the title of Lance Armstrong's book, *It's Not About the Bike*. For me, it was all about the bike! His ability to shift his focus from cancer back to his bike set a glaring example for me. It's really a common thread in all cancer survivor stories. There is some point at which we survivors patiently and gradually change our focus.

I remember reading a book by Cheryl Canfield titled *Profound Healing*. Although I read it many years ago, Cheryl's story still inspires me. Here was a woman who was dying and there was no denying that fact. She couldn't afford treatment. She was alone and just trying to find a way to die with dignity. The way she approached this daunting task was by going within. Her search to find the good qualities within herself eventually led to her healing. It's an amazing story. On the surface, her focus was to find a way to come to terms with death and dying. Her journey involved reviewing everything in her life, including all the people who'd caused her great pain and anger. She addressed each painful situation and the people involved in great detail. Hers is a story anyone can relate to with much heartache and emotion. She started journaling and even wrote letters of forgiveness. She not only found ways to face these issues, she found ways to release them with love and discovery of a new perspective. This book made me realize how much pain and hurt we humans suppress and never really face head on. We ignore and we become ill. In the beginning, her intention was to die with dignity, but at some point her focus shifted to forgiveness and letting go. I interpreted her journey as one that wasn't so much about dying as it was about her intention of coming to terms with her life.

The power of intention is undeniable. If you haven't been exposed to Dr. Wayne W. Dyer's work, then you have no idea what you're missing. This man is incredible and amazing. I have purchased many of his CDs and books. I've also watched him on public television. I highly recommend his books and audiotapes or CDs. They can change your life. It is impossible to write a chapter on focus without mentioning experts like Dr. Dyer, Louise L. Hay, Caroline Myss and Eckhart Tolle. These are just a few of the wonderful people whose compelling words can genuinely help guide you in your healing. Your focus and your intentions are powerful beyond belief. We are lucky to live in a time and place where this valuable knowledge is available to all. These gifted people remind us of our value, power and purpose.

As you go through your day, pay close attention to your thoughts. Make it your intention to focus on the wonderful things life has to offer. Be grateful and loving. Even if this is your last day on earth, let it be a day that pleases you right down to your soul.

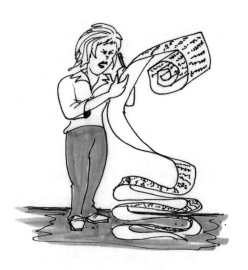

Inventory

When I was diagnosed with recurring ovarian cancer, I really had a difficult time comprehending why the cancer returned. I was eating healthy, getting plenty of fresh air and exercise and I wasn't smoking, drinking or anything like that. In fact, I didn't even have job-related stress because it had been years since I'd worked. Plus, I had a history of health and well-being prior to the arrival of cancer in 2000.

I couldn't understand why this was happening. Just what was going on with me, anyway? Why was my immune system compromised? This got me thinking. Perhaps my immune system was so busy doing other things that there was nothing left for battling cancer. After my third surgery and completing another six months of chemotherapy, I decided to take more responsibility for myself and that meant taking a close look at what I was exposing myself to.

I started by taking an inventory of everything I put on my body or in my mouth. The first thing I did every morning was brush my teeth. So I wrote down all the ingredients in my toothpaste. I wondered, "Why is my toothpaste made of all chemicals?" Of all the ingredients in my toothpaste, the only ones I recognized didn't seem healthy; such as blue and yellow dye. There was also sodium, saccharin and glycerin. What about the fluoride? What is fluoride, anyway? Let me assure you, once you do some research on fluoride, you'll never feel safe about fluoride again. Well, this was no way to start my day!

Next, I jumped in the shower. Without much thought, I lathered up the old body with soap and cleaned my hair using my favorite shampoo and conditioner. Once I was out and dried off, I wrote down all the ingredients in those items. Again, I found myself stunned by the list of ingredients. Not only did I not recognize any of the ingredients, there were so many of them! It was frightening. I could just imagine myself going into a store and asking, "Where's the titanium dioxide and petrolatuim?" I'm sure people would think I was nuts, but there they were – and many more chemicals. They were right there in the products I put on my body. I was afraid to go further with my morning routine, but I knew it was something I had to do.

I reluctantly pulled out the lotion that I'd normally slather all over my body. This time I read the ingredients before I applied it to my skin. Sure enough, the list of chemicals was dizzying. Forget about using body lotion today. I moved on to my deodorant and wondered why I needed to put all those chemicals under my arms where there are so many lymph nodes and so close to my breasts. I recognized aluminum there on the list – why was aluminum in my underarm deodorant? I dreaded the next step – applying my cosmetics. Oh, what a list of crap I had already accumulated and I hadn't even put any breakfast in my mouth yet. Then came the hair styling products. Should I use mousse or gel today? Oh, and don't forget the hair spray. By the time I made it downstairs to the kitchen, I already felt depressed.

I could tell it was time to take some responsibility for what happened to my body. I might not be able to control everything, but surely I could do something about the products I chose to use. I know the FDA and other important government agencies say that these ingredients are safe, but are they really safe? Maybe a little bit of aluminum in my deodorant was safe, but when you add it to the aluminum in my body lotion, my cosmetics – and what about the aluminum I get from my cookware or if I broil something on aluminum foil? Is it still a safe amount then? By the end of the day, the "little bit of aluminum" could turn into a lot.

Once you count up all the chemicals and toxins you put on your body throughout the day, it's one big toxic festival. I hadn't even eaten yet and I had already exposed my poor immune system to hundreds of toxins. I wondered if I could find products that were healthy and safe. After all, if I could eliminate hundreds of toxins simply by changing some of the products I used, maybe I could give my poor immune system a break. It was something to consider.

Downstairs, it was time for breakfast. I fixed a scrambled egg, toast with margarine and poured some orange juice. Well, here we go. I'd thought this was a pretty healthy breakfast until I started writing down the ingredients.

Why does everything have to have so much crap in it? Is it simply for profit? Is it processed with all these chemicals and preservatives in order to keep it on the store shelves for months at a time? I was frustrated. Here I thought I was being healthy. There are so many ingredients in margarine that the list wraps around the entire lid! What happened to real food? The bread didn't seem much better. Lots of questionable ingredients there, too. I went through the day and listed all the ingredients in everything I ate, drank and put on my body. By the end of the day, I had exposed myself to thousands of chemicals and toxins. The worst part was that these were my personal choices. No one else was responsible for what I put on and in my body. That responsibility fell directly on my shoulders.

At first, I felt helpless. It seemed overwhelming. What could I do about it? There were chemicals and toxins everywhere and in everything. You know, my life was so much easier when I expected someone else to fix me. I could sit back, have operations followed by chemo and someone else could be responsible for my health. Well, sorry lady, but it just doesn't work that way. I had to face reality. If my immune system was compromised, I sure hadn't helped it out. It felt like a bomb had been dropped on me. I now knew what most people don't want to know. Okay, I wanted to bury my head in the sand and pretend these things didn't make a difference in my health, but that was a lie and my intuition wouldn't let it go. I had to do something.

Since I felt so overwhelmed, I decided it was best to slow down and take this one step at a time. I decided I'd start with my regular shopping. As I replenished items, I would make new choices – one product at a time. I reminded myself that even if I replaced one toxic product with a new wholesome choice, it would result in eliminating probably twenty or more chemical toxins. I stayed encouraged by realizing that even one small change makes a difference. So if I couldn't find the right product this time, I didn't freak out, I simply kept looking. I found many products at Whole Foods Market and many on the Internet. And now, even my local market carries organic foods. It got to the point where shopping became an adventure. It was no longer work. I admit there was a lot of trial and error. I found products that were pure, but they didn't work to my satisfaction. What good is chemical-free laundry soap if your clothes still look dirty? In the end, it wasn't that difficult to find great laundry soap. I also stopped using chemical dryer sheets. What sense does it make to use toxin-free detergent, only to turn around and throw a bunch of chemicals on your clothes with dryer sheets?

Keep in mind that anything you put on your skin is absorbed into your body via your bloodstream. If you don't believe it, think for a minute. Instead of taking a pill, you can now use a patch. These patches administer substances into your bloodstream through your skin. There are nicotine patches, hormone patches and more. So what you put on your clothes and bedding is important. Since your skin touches your clothes throughout the day and your bedding during the night, you don't want toxins on these items. As it turns out, there are plenty of natural products available. The more toxins you can eliminate, the better. The way I figure it, if I eliminate toxins, then my immune system doesn't have to do it for me. As far as I'm concerned, my immune system needs to pay attention to more critical things.

What were all these chemicals, anyway? I read the labels, but it was as though I was reading some other language.

Basically, I stayed with products that listed ingredients I understood. If I didn't know what an ingredient was, I passed on buying that item. I really wanted to know an easy way to interpret labels. I wanted to make better choices and I wanted to obtain knowledge that could help me. Eventually, the best information about understanding labels came from Kevin Trudeau's book and CDs, *Natural Cures 'They' Don't Want You to Know About*. His information about reading food labels was particularly alarming but at least I knew the truth and I could see I was on the right track with my approach to all these products and foods. There's nothing like knowledge when it comes to labels. Kevin Trudeau helped me see even more areas where I could improve in my purchases. This information actually helped me expand my food and product choices. Once I understood labels, I found lots of healthy items. Thank you, Kevin!

I'm somewhat dumbfounded at the way the majority of people respond to this topic. It's bad enough that most healthy people think it's a bunch of nonsense, but when people have serious illnesses, they still brush it aside. People say, "I can't change my diet," or "The government wouldn't allow it if it wasn't safe." The truth is that most people have become so lazy that they simply don't want to change anything about their lifestyles. It's sad. Most people think it's too difficult to change, but it isn't. It's easy.

If you can read, then what could be difficult about reading a label? You'll be surprised at how easy it is to differentiate food words from chemical and food additive words. Select foods by the ingredients on the labels. If you don't recognize an ingredient as food, simply stop putting it in your mouth. If you can't find organic wholesome foods, then change where you shop. You're the one who decides what goes in your mouth to feed your body. Food choices are your responsibility and your personal contribution to your current state of health and healing.

People find lots of excuses for not taking responsibility for their health. I'm no different. I had all the excuses. The main excuses are time and convenience. People say they don't have time to eat healthy, so they hit the drive-through at a fast food restaurant. And they say there's no time for exercise because, "I can't miss my favorite television program." There's always the money excuse. That's a big one. I often hear people say it costs too much to purchase healthy products. I'm here to tell you about the one thing that trumps them all. Illness is never cheap or convenient. Have you ever thought about how much money it costs to get sick? If you don't have time to take care of yourself now, what will you do when a serious illness strikes? It's not easy, either. There's nothing convenient, quick or simple when it comes to cancer treatments. If you think you can't afford to buy healthy products, wait until you see the bill for cancer!

There's no better place to start than by taking an inventory of the products you consume and use on your body. It is truly a reality check. I think everyone can benefit by doing this at least once. You can and should participate in your healing. Start taking responsiblity for yourself. It may take some extra time to read labels when you're shopping. I admit I do most of my shopping where I know the foods are organic and/or locally grown. It's true that this isn't as convenient as going down the street to the local market, but it's worth it. And before you know it, you'll find it's enjoyable to spend extra time on enhancing your health.

If you really want to do something that has a positive impact on your health, I believe this is the main thing you can do. It doesn't matter what type of illness you're dealing with – eliminating toxins is key. Don't be afraid of what others think or say. This is your life and it is precious. Hold yourself accountable. You are the one who decides what you put in your mouth and on your body. Be proud of your choices. Your body will thank you and the results will astound you.

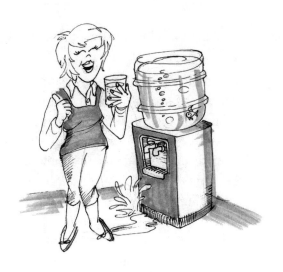

Water

Y ou may want to begin with drinking more clean, uncontaminated water. This is one of the easiest things
you can do to improve your life. If there is nothing else you
can do at this moment, then water is a good place to start.
Drinking lots of water will help eliminate toxins and keep
you hydrated. Although you can live quite a while without
food, water is a different story. You must have water in order to survive and to maintain good health. Every cell in
your body needs water. It is required for nourishment and
for eliminating waste.

Drinking more water sounds simple enough, yet there
are some real concerns about the quality of the water we
drink. I think the most valuable information I learned about
water came from Dr. Hulda Clark, author of several books
including, *The Cure for All Cancers*. I highly recommend
Dr. Clark's books. Not only will you learn more about the

importance of water, you'll learn many other common things that affect your health and healing.

Many people feel that drinking tap water is out of the question, yet Dr. Clark presents an interesting perspective on this topic. She feels that drinking tap water may not be a bad idea at all. Of course, that depends on the conditions of your tap water. It is a constantly available and flowing source of water, which is good. You certainly don't want to drink water that is stagnant. It is crucial that your tap water is not contaminated. It is also very important that the pipes in your home are not corroded or leaching metals into the water. You can always have your water tested to ensure it is safe for drinking. I was surprised to hear that Dr. Clark found many areas with safe tap water. The opinion of some, including our water company, is that drinking tap water may be safe.

According to Dr. Clark, Dr. Jennifer Brett and many others, the best and least expensive way to drink safe water is by using activated carbon or charcoal filters. The carbon filter removes most of the carcinogens and bacteria commonly found in drinking water. These filters are inexpensive and you can find them in most department stores or on the Internet. If you have any doubt about the water you are consuming, this would be the best way to approach it quickly and easily, with little cost.

I understand that Dr. Clark has made some new discoveries regarding chlorine in water and its effect on our bodies. I recently learned she has developed a water filtration system that comes with pre-washed activated charcoal from coconut shells. It removes nearly all organic and volatile organic chemical contaminants and removes more than 99 percent of the chlorine. You can obtain information on this new system by visiting www.drclarkuniversity.org. It is always interesting to learn about Dr. Clark's discoveries.

Many people have water filtration or purification systems installed in their homes. This requires some research. The water purification system I had in my home when I was diagnosed with cancer was a soft water system that required putting salt in the system periodically. Softener salts are polluted with strontium and chromate. They are also full of aluminum. The water softener salts corrode the pipes, then the pipes begin to seep cadmium into the water. I'm not saying that system gave me cancer, but I removed it as quickly as possible. This type of soft water system is now outlawed in many areas. That fact alone led me to believe it was not contributing to my good health! Shortly after we removed that system, our hot water heater needed to be replaced. I'm glad we replaced it, too. The water heater was corroded and contaminated after years of soft water running through it. It wasn't until we replaced the water filtration system and the hot water heater that the tap water finally tested clean and pure.

While I was looking for a replacement water system for our home, my husband suggested that I contact what he referred to as one of his "touchy-feely" clients. He said they were awesome people; into the holistic thing and I'd like them. Sure enough, it was through these folks that we purchased our Life Source home water system. They explained why activated carbon systems are safe and healthy. It was good reinforcement for me, since Dr. Clark had stressed the same things when I was under her care. I felt so much better knowing I wasn't being sold just any system. I learned the important differences in water and its impact on our bodies. There is plenty of information available about drinking water and why soft water is not for drinking. So if you are sick and have a soft water system in your home as I did, you will surely want to research the pros and cons of drinking soft water.

My concern with water isn't just about drinking it. Remember that you bathe in it, wash your clothes and dishes in it and cook with it. Your skin is your largest organ and everything you put on your skin gets absorbed into your bloodstream. This is why I feel it's very important to have pure, clean water in my home. I often enjoy soaking in a hot bath, but when I don't have time for a bath, I still shower daily. My body absorbs a lot of water every day – so the cleaner, the better!

Obviously, not everyone can afford to purchase a home water filtration system, but you can make sure to drink plenty of good, clean water every day. Many people insist on only bottled water. There are pros and cons on this topic as well. Dr. Clark reports that bottled water often has isopropyl alcohol in it as part of the way the bottles are cleaned before they're filled. Dr. Clark's findings show that all cancer patients have isopropyl alcohol in their systems. Perhaps the isopropyl alcohol contributes to cancer or perhaps because we have cancer, our compromised immune systems aren't able to eliminate this toxin. Dr. Day reports that she knows of people who have gotten better while drinking bottled water. There are many types of bottled water – spring water, Kabbalah water (prayed over by rabbis), purified water, flavored water and more.

There are also many proponents of distilled water. You can purchase systems for distilling water in your home and distilled water is available in stores. I would advise you to approach this with caution. There is a tremendous amount of literature available that tells of the problems associated with drinking distilled water. It actually leaches minerals from your body. There is also a correlation between consuming soft water (distilled water is soft) and cardiovascular disease. While distilled water may be beneficial for a short detoxification period of a few weeks, it usually proves dangerous in the end. According to Zoltan P. Rona, MD, MSc, "Longevity is associated with the regular consumption of hard water" (high in minerals).

Your water preference, like all things, is a personal choice based on your own interpretation of the information available. One thing is certain, though; we all need water to survive. If you are currently ill and are still drinking sodas or soft drinks, I recommend that you eliminate them completely. Replace those liquids with good, clean water. You will be doing your body a great favor. Remember the significance of small steps. Even something as small as this one step – switching to good, clean water – can make a wonderful difference in your health. It is surprising how your body responds when you replace toxic chemical-laden drinks with good, clean water.

Recently, I learned about the groundbreaking work being done by Masaru Emoto, an internationally renowned Japanese researcher. His *New York Times* Bestseller, *The Hidden Messages in Water*, is astounding. Emoto's research findings stunned me. I found it hard to believe what I read. His research provides evidence that thoughts, music, words and ideas affect the molecular structure of water. Emoto's water crystallization photographs demonstrate how water forms beautiful delicate crystals when exposed to classical and other beautiful music. In contrast, the water formed fragmented and malformed crystals when exposed to violent heavy metal music. It doesn't stop there.

When Emoto experimented with words or phrases, the results were just as amazing. He wrapped pieces of paper with words such as "thank you" and "fool" around bottles of water, with the words facing into the water. The water that was exposed to "thank you" formed gorgeous hexagonal crystals, while the water exposed to the word "fool" created malformed and fragmented crystals. His photographs of water exposed to the words "You Make Me Sick. I Will Kill You" and water exposed to the words of a deceased killer's name – Adolph Hitler – resulted in ugly, distorted shapes.

I was most impacted by photographs of water before and after prayer. What a difference! There were photos of water from the Fujiwara Dam, Lake Zurich and The Bahamas – even plain old tap water. All showed undeniable and remarkable differences, before and after. And they were not small changes. They were striking and incredibly beautiful transformations.

Emoto speaks of the power of love and gratitude. These two words, used together, formed the most beautiful crystals. The word "love" alone formed beautiful crystals, but when combined with the word "gratitude," the crystals that formed showed a remarkable depth and refinement, a diamond-like brilliance. Whether you use words, music, prayers or intentions, the molecular structure of water reacts. Now think about your body.

Your body is seventy percent water – and water covers seventy percent of our planet. You have to wonder if that is a coincidence. What are your thoughts, words, emotions and intentions doing to your body – or for that matter to the waters of the world? Now I focus on thinking, feeling and reflecting often on love and gratitude. I realize the vital effect it has on my body and on my healing.

Emoto's work is far too valuable to overlook or disregard. Some might say it's all a bunch of hogwash, but please do yourself a favor and make up your own mind. Information about Masaru Emoto and his research is abundant. He has written several books and gives lectures throughout the world. My first encounter with his work occurred when I watched the DVD, *What the Bleep!? Down the Rabbit Hole.* You can also learn more about the validity of his work through doing some research of your own on the Internet.

After reading Emoto's research about prayer, it made me think there just might be something to that Kabbalah water that the celebrities are drinking lately. After all, it is prayed over by rabbis. Actually, Emoto's research changed my thinking about a lot of things. I have a feeling it will change your thinking, too. So, if you're interested, you can find a wealth of information about how important water is to your health and healing.

My point is that in order to get healthy and stay healthy, you need to drink plenty of clean, uncontaminated water. If you are sick, it may be worth it to take a closer look at the source of water you drink. The most important thing to remember is that we all must have water in order to survive. The quality of that water is crucial and it does impact your health and healing. Please drink plenty of clean water!

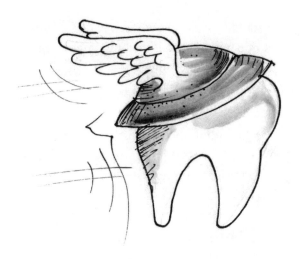

Chew on This

I've discovered lots of information since I decided to reclaim my health, but none more disturbing than the connection between dentistry and illness. Like most people, I assumed that dental products and materials were completely safe. It was absurd to think otherwise…or was it?

The more I read, the angrier I became. Amalgam fillings are commonly called "silver" fillings. They should be called mercury fillings, because they are approximately fifty percent mercury. Oh, and there's other metal in amalgam fillings, too. Metals such as tin, silver, copper and sometimes even nickel! The fact that each filling is about fifty percent mercury truly floored me. Mercury is poisonous!

They tell pregnant women not to eat fish because of mercury, but no one says anything about the mercury we suck on all day and all night from our own teeth! It's no secret that mercury and other metals slowly leak from fillings. Furthermore, mercury can actually vaporize when it leaves a filling. When this happens, we inhale it and our lungs immediately absorb mercury. This can happen any time, but it's worse when we eat or chew. Mercury is one of the most toxic of all metals and it doesn't belong in our bodies.

If you think small amounts of mercury aren't anything to worry about, pay close attention. Mercury is so toxic that any mercury filling material left after a tooth is filled is considered toxic waste and must be disposed of according to strict Environmental Protection Agency (EPA) guidelines. It is against the law to put any mercury filling material into a landfill. If mercury can poison a landfill, it certainly doesn't belong in your mouth. Mercury poisons every cell it enters. It is so toxic that mercury clean-up efforts are taking place worldwide. I read that the amount of mercury on a pinhead, once airborne, is enough to cause a fish advisory on a forty-acre lake. After seeing that, it was no surprise to learn that there is a genuine concern about crematoriums. The air pollution caused by burning bodies with amalgam fillings is a real issue. Mercury is an element; that means it cannot be broken down into other components. That's why it is almost impossible to get rid of mercury once it has entered the environment.

If mercury is that toxic, why is there mercury in our so-called "silver" fillings? Do you realize that your dentist cannot give you your extracted tooth if that tooth contains a silver filling? Apparently, it's too dangerous for you to put your own tooth in your pocket and take it home. In one breath, they tell you the tooth is safe in your mouth, yet in the next breath, they tell you it's dangerous once outside your mouth and you can't take it home. How stupid do they think we are? Apparently, we are plenty stupid, because amalgam fillings are still used daily. And this information isn't anything new.

The federal government and the American Dental Association (ADA) are well aware of the poisonous effects of inhaling mercury from dental fillings. Mercury is the most toxic non-radioactive element on the planet. While most medical and scientific researchers have called for a ban on the use of mercury in all products, our government chooses to ignore it when it comes to dentistry. I know that if you followed the money trail, it would become obvious why this danger is ignored.

Long-term exposure to mercury results in plenty of illnesses. Depression, birth defects, kidney problems, heart damage, memory loss and many more health problems can be directly related to mercury poisoning. In a book titled *Tooth Truth*, author Frank Jerome, DDS explains how mercury particularly likes nerve cells, including those in the brain. Dr. Jerome points out that mercury attacks the nervous system. This should be a serious concern for people with multiple sclerosis (MS), Alzheimer's disease and Parkinson's disease. The book is filled with valuable information and should be a must-read for anyone with silver fillings – even those who aren't yet sick.

The mercury in your dental fillings has been shown to adversely affect your body's immune response and that is a major concern for people dealing with cancer. In fact, a dental clean-up may be one of the most important steps you can take when it comes to healing yourself. In fact, it's the first step required to be one of Dr. Hulda Clark's patients. I had my dental clean-up during the short period of time I spent under her care.

I first learned the frightening truth about mercury fillings through reading Dr. Clark's books. That led me to *Tooth Truth*, mentioned above. *Tooth Truth* led me to *It's All In Your Head*, by Dr. Hal A. Huggins. From there, I went to the Internet, where I learned how silver fillings are disposed of in my area. I found lots of information about how we get mercury poisoning from fillings and more. If you're looking for a dentist who doesn't use mercury fillings or someone who can properly remove the mercury from your mouth, check the Internet.

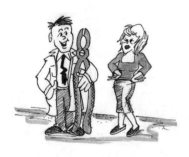

When I learned that all my mercury fillings had to go, I felt good and bad at the same time. I'd read case after case of people who'd conquered debilitating illnesses simply by having their fillings removed. Those accounts made me feel good. Going to the dentist and dealing with my teeth, however, made me feel bad! But it had to be done. There are plenty of other dental materials available and many are biocompatible (non-toxic). There's just no reason for you to have mercury in your mouth. It's a cumulative poison, so the longer you have it in your mouth, the more damage it can do. Once your fillings are removed, it will take time for your body to detoxify. It can take a month for every year you've had your fillings – and it may be impossible to eliminate the mercury from every cell. The sooner you get rid of your "silver" fillings, the better off you'll be.

Information about "silver" fillings and illness is abundant. What I've mentioned here is only the tip of the iceberg.

And don't even get me started on fluoride! That's another poison we are over-exposed to, thanks to the ADA. Please do yourself a favor. Read these books and do some research. I promise you won't regret it.

I hope I have raised your curiosity enough that you will do some research for yourself. Don't take your dentist's word that these mercury-filled materials are safe – because *they are not safe*. They are not safe for you, your children or anyone else. Once you know the truth, you can help spread the word. The sooner people are informed, the faster we can eliminate this horrible and deadly practice.

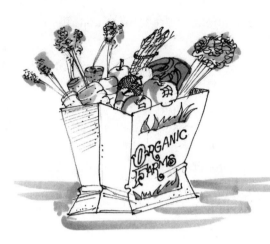

Let's Eat

Let's talk about food. Most of us enjoy eating delicious food, but how does food impact health? I was surprised to learn that diet has a lot to do with health, especially when it comes to cancer.

I'd always had a good appetite. I thought I ate a well-balanced diet with plenty of vegetables. So what was the problem? Part of the problem was that I'd based my belief system on old patterns. I still used the old food group chart from school. I quickly learned the food pyramid from my youth was outdated and no longer considered a healthy way to eat. That was the first surprise. Many more followed.

At first, I didn't think my research on nutrition would result in more than a few minor changes in my eating habits. After all, how hard could it be to follow the new food pyramid? As I read more, I wondered if the changes would really be that simple. The more I learned, the more suspicious I became about the recommendations on the new food pyramid.

The first changes I made were a result of a couple of videos by Lorraine Day, MD – *Cancer Doesn't Scare Me Anymore* and *You Can't Improve On God*. In these videos, Dr. Day shares her cancer survival story. She even includes photographs of the tumor protruding from her chest. Doctors told her she was going to die, but she didn't! Let me tell you, hers is an incredible story. She's the one who got me started on the right path when it comes to food choices. It's very hard to ignore someone like Dr. Day, who is first and foremost a true cancer survivor. Her credentials are also impeccable.

Dr. Day is an internationally acclaimed orthopedic trauma surgeon and she is recognized worldwide as an AIDS expert. She was chief of orthopedic surgery at San Francisco General Hospital and her credentials go on and on. Need I say more? I received more education and insight about cancer, diet and food from her videos than I ever dreamed possible. Do yourself a favor and visit her web site at www. drday.com.

I'd like to recommend two other books that had a great impact in teaching me the importance of food choices: *The pH Miracle*, by Robert O. Young, PhD and Shelley Redford Young and *Natural Cures 'They' Don't Want You To Know About*, by Kevin Trudeau.

I could list more resources, but I limited myself to those that provided me with the most value. With so much out there in the way of books, reports and the Internet, it's easy to get overwhelmed with too much information. These two resources provide a quick and easy understanding of why and how dietary changes have such a tremendous impact when it comes to changing the course of deadly diseases.

Since ovarian cancer certainly falls into the category of one of the deadliest diseases, I figured I'd better pay attention. I'd had a wake-up call. I knew I had to make dietary changes if survival was my true goal. I'll admit I don't follow any one diet to perfection, but I sure set high standards. There are always times when we cannot control the circumstances. The same is true with food. If I'm eating out or in someone's home, my food choices may be limited. However, I still make a conscious effort to select the most appropriate foods available.

The one place I have complete control is in my home. This is where great strides pay off. I figure that I eat at home eighty to ninety percent of the time. So my home contains food I choose. Almost everything I buy is organic. And there's more to organic food than I first thought. Before my illness, I thought organically grown food was simply food that wasn't sprayed with pesticides. I thought that if I washed it thoroughly, that would rid the food of toxins. I was wrong. I learned that conventionally grown food is grown in soil that is so toxic that even earthworms can't live in it. That scared me. If the soil is filled with chemicals, fertilizers and other toxins, surely these will somehow end up in the food. I didn't want that stuff to end up inside me, so organic food was a simple choice.

I thought it would be difficult to find organically grown food, but I was pleasantly surprised. I started by doing my grocery shopping at the Whole Foods Market, where they clearly label produce as organically grown or conventionally grown. That made shopping easy. I found all sorts of organic food there. Everything from milk to bread and nuts to sauces – all were available in organic. A new healthy world opened up for me. Just by marketing at Whole Foods, life became much simpler. Just recently, my local Vons Market started carrying organic products, too. While the selection isn't as good as at Whole Foods, it is improving. And it's so convenient. When I only need a few items for a fresh salad or some organic fruit, I just run down the street instead of making the longer trip through traffic to Whole Foods. These days, you'll notice more organic products showing up on your supermarket shelves, too.

For the most part, I eat a vegetarian diet. On rare occasions, I allow myself to eat meat or poultry, but never pork. It's important to me that the animal was raised without hormones or antibiotics. So far, I've only found this available at Whole Foods Market or through Suzanne Somers' infomercials. I'm sure there are many other places to purchase this type of meat, but since I've essentially eliminated it from my diet; I just haven't looked. Dr. Day gave me enough incentive for eliminating meat. After watching her videos, I realized just how crucial it was for beating this disease. Like I said, I'm not perfect, but it's uncommon for me to eat meat or poultry.

I do enjoy fish, mostly salmon, but even that isn't part of my normal diet. I prefer to keep to a vegetarian plan, organic of course. Eating lots of vegetables keeps your body in an alkaline, rather than acidic, state. When your body is in an acidic state, it is vulnerable to germs. I'm no expert, but you can learn more in *The pH Miracle*. I often make salad dressing out of flaxseed oil or even fish oil that includes omega-3s and omega-6s. Add some lemon juice and spices and it's as simple as that. These fats strengthen cell walls and they strengthen your immune system. You can also buy pre-made organic salad dressing or you may prefer to make your own.

The most important thing about eating healthy and organic is eliminating toxins. The more toxins you can eliminate from your body, the better off you'll be. After I learned how to read labels, I was stunned by the number of chemicals and toxins that are disguised as words such as "spices" and "flavors." Kevin Trudeau's book armed me with real knowledge about how to read food labels. With this information alone, I eliminated hundreds of chemicals from my diet. It's frightening to learn how many toxins we are exposed to through our food. It's scary because it almost seems to have been done intentionally at some levels. Intentional or not, we must deal with it. The best thing to do is to get back to a balanced, natural and organic diet.

Most of us don't pay attention to the amount of dye contained in food. You just assume that everything in your food is safe. Unfortunately, that's a dangerous assumption. While a little dye in one product may be safe, what happens when you add up all the dye in all the products you consume on a daily basis? Is it still safe then? By day's end, it's no longer a small amount. There's even dye in toothpaste! It is important to avoid food that contains dye. Dye is not healthy and it is very difficult to eliminate dye from your body. Check the label – you'll be amazed to find out how much dye is contained in the products you consume.

Most over-the-counter pain relievers are coated with dye. Next time you decide to take one of those colorful pills, run it under some water and use your fingers to rub the dye off the pill before you take it. You'll be amazed when you see the amount of dye on just one pill. You'll also see how difficult it is to get the dye off your fingers. It isn't hard to imagine how difficult it is for your body to get rid of this dye.

Think about how much dye was on that one pill. Then consider that it's only one small source of all the dye you ingest daily. Many products contain dye and your body has to work hard to get rid of it. If you are ill, is this a task you want your body to work on? Or would you prefer that your body work on more important tasks, such as fighting your disease? Pay attention to your shopping choices, particularly when it comes to food.

Sticking to a new eating routine isn't as difficult as you might think. You'll find that natural food actually tastes better and your food cravings will change. Just because you're eating healthy, it doesn't mean you have to sacrifice delicious foods. I still love waking up to the smell of coffee in the morning. Even though coffee might not be on the list of healthy choices, I don't feel guilty about my morning coffee because now it is organic – not laden with pesticides.

Balance is the key to good health. They say everything in moderation, but there are some things you should avoid at all costs.

Cross fast food restaurants off your list completely. The food has been processed and loaded with empty calories. Get off of artificial sweeteners and white sugar, too. There are alternatives, such as honey and agava nectar. Do a little research and you'll be surprised. There's always a healthy alternative.

I avoid soft drinks completely and you should, too. There is nothing healthy about canned or bottled soft drinks.

It makes no difference if they contain sugar or if they are sugar-fee. Avoid them at all costs. For me, water is the only choice. I do drink organic juice and love fresh-squeezed juice. Buy a juicer and make the most of it. It's a wonderful way to get lots of healthy nutrients. You can juice fruit and vegetables. Look at Jack LaLanne – what an amazing role model. He is a proponent of juicing and you just can't argue when you see how it's paid off for him. I also enjoy tea. Some of my favorites are green, black and ginseng tea.

Another way I get lots of nutrients is by consuming green drinks. Green drinks contain the nutritional benefits of green plants and vegetables often lacking in our diets. It's important that the green drink you choose is organic. You wouldn't want to get a concentrate of pesticides along with all those wonderful nutrients. There are plenty to choose from; just make sure anything you choose is organic. Another benefit is the alkalizing effect green drinks have on the body. I even put pH drops in my drinking water to ensure I keep myself in a more alkaline, rather than acidic, state. Keeping your body alkaline is important when it comes to great health. There are lots of pH drops available on the Internet.

Nuts and seeds are my favorites, too. I particularly enjoy them when they're raw and organic. While many people fear the high calorie content, I don't pay attention to it. I eat nuts by the handful and it hasn't affected my weight. Perhaps it's because I've eliminated so much processed food that's high in empty calories and unhealthy fats.

You may think converting to organic food won't go over with the rest of your family, but this just isn't true. My family had been eating organic food when they visited my home long before I told them about my converting to organic. In fact, I often got compliments about the delicious meals I fixed. Even picky eaters eat well at my home, including my two-year-old grandson! I've found organic products such as macaroni and cheese, lemonade, popcorn, pancake mix and many other things the children enjoy. They eat organic fruit, vegetables and dairy products. When someone offers food to my seven-year-old grandson, it's cute to hear him ask, "Is it organic?" I've been able to convert my family's favorite recipes entirely to organic. I feel good knowing that the food they get at Grandma's house is clean and healthy.

Each of these little things adds up to big gains when it comes to fighting a life-threatening disease. Food is meant to nourish your body; not just satisfy your hunger. There were times when I was very strict about my food choices, sticking closely to the pH diet or following Dr. Day's diet without exception. When I regained my energy and had strengthened my immune system, I relaxed and allowed myself to eat small amounts of dairy, fish and now I even drink coffee.

Now that I have regained my health, I no longer have to be a fanatic about everything. I know in my heart that my home is a safe haven. I spend the majority of my time living and eating at home. To me that means when I go out or have dinner at a friend's house, I can relax and enjoy it. My body is now in a state that it can handle an occasional meal that may not be organic. I feel I can have a glass of wine or a cocktail once in a while. Since I've made these important changes in my eating habits, I haven't looked back. The rewards are far too great. While I may not be perfect, I don't feel guilty having a little ice cream or birthday cake when the occasion arises.

I don't expect others to conform to my lifestyle and I'm not saying it's the right choice for you. However, I do believe it is absolutely necessary to eliminate needless chemicals and toxins from our food. I feel this is critical. It seems to me that my poor immune system was frazzled just trying to keep up with eliminating my daily intake of thousands of chemicals. It didn't have anything left to fight my serious illness. That's why I changed my diet. I hope this will inspire you to look closely at your food choices as part of your journey to healing. Remember, it's the little things that add up to great improvements.

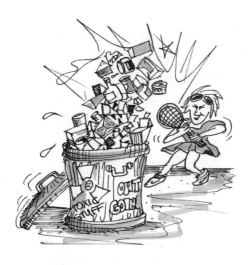

Kitchen Habits

M y kitchen habits changed dramatically as a result of research done by Dr. Hulda Clark. According to Dr. Clark, all cancer patients – that's one hundred percent of us – have both isopropyl alcohol and the intestinal fluke parasite in our livers. You can read more of Dr. Clark's cancer research in any of her books. She has cured many cancer patients without surgery, radiation or chemotherapy. Whether you agree with her theories or not, don't ignore her kitchen and food recommendations.

Before you do anything else, make sure you remove all the toxic items from your kitchen. You need to do this throughout your home, but the kitchen is an absolute must! Anything that contains chemicals and is stored under the kitchen sink or in a cabinet needs to be removed and put in the garage or the garbage. This means any type of chemical cleaners, floor wax, furniture polish, roach and ant killers –

anything with chemicals must go. Your kitchen needs to be safe. Toxic chemicals just do not belong in the kitchen where you prepare and cook food. It just makes sense.

I now prepare food in glass, ceramic or microwavable cookware. The microwave oven is my last choice when it comes to preparing food. My grandson Mason and I did an experiment Kevin Trudeau recommends. We planted the exact same number and type of seeds in separate pots. We used the same soil and seed source. We gave each the same amount of water and sun. The only difference was one pot got water from the stovetop (heated then cooled) and the other from the microwave (also heated and cooled). The seeds given stovetop water produced far more plants than the seeds that got microwave water – and they were healthier, too. We decided that microwaving isn't as healthy as heating from the stovetop. That's why the microwave oven is my last choice for preparing food.

If you use a pressure cooker, as I do from time to time, put the food in a glass bowl with a lid that fits inside the pressure cooker. Also, do not use any special spray to grease pans; that spray contains silicone.

You should try to reduce your contact with metal as much as possible. I use my crock pot several times during the week to prepare meals. I also use plastic or wooden utensils for cooking. I got rid of most of my metal utensils long ago. I tried to use plastic knives for food preparation, but I just couldn't deal with it. I have a wonderful set of Cutco knives that makes preparing food much easier.

When I'm at home, I don't eat with silverware or flatware. I use plastic cutlery. It's not the type you get with take-out foods or the kind you buy for birthday parties. I use a sturdier type for camping and backpacking that I found at a local sporting goods store. It's even dishwasher safe. While my family prefers to use regular flatware, I always eat with the plastic ware at home. I have to agree with Dr. Clark, who says, "Stop sucking on metal lollipops!"

Dr. Clark reminds us that most stainless steel cookware contains eighteen percent chromium and eight percent nickel. Just because you can't see the metal deteriorating, don't think it isn't happening. Dr. Clark emphasizes that all metal seeps. So get rid of your metal pots. I believe that getting your iron from spinach is far safer than getting it from a cast-iron pan. There is one exception – stainless steel 18/10. Dr. Clark recently discovered that this particular type of stainless steel cookware is so hard that it doesn't leach nickel, chromium, iron and some other metals. Be careful when shopping, though, because it's easy to mistake 18/0 for 18/10. Another important thing: I know how much we all love our coated pans because nothing sticks to them and they're so easy to clean, but Dr. Clark doesn't recommend them and neither do I. If you doubt their toxicity, here's something to think about.

My friend Michele loves parrots and all types of birds. She had her last three birds for many years and they were a precious part of her family. One day after recovering from the flu, Michele finally felt like she could eat something. She went to the stove and put a non-stick coated pan on the burner to heat, then left the room for a minute while the pan was heating. She got distracted for ten minutes or so and suddenly realized she'd forgotten the pan heating on the stove. As she entered the room, she noticed her parrot was barely standing. She looked over at the parakeets.

One was already dead and the other one was fading fast. Panicked and confused as to what could be going on, she rushed the birds out to the fresh air. She quickly realized it must be the empty pan heating on the stove. She removed the pan. There was no smoke coming from it. It didn't appear to have any damage at all. The pan was still intact, yet her beloved birds were now dead. You can only imagine how devastated she was. For days, she could barely talk. She felt awful; it was as if she had murdered her own birds. That was two years ago and she still can't bring herself to get another bird. Michele thought, "If heating a pan with non-stick coating can kill my birds that quickly, what is it doing to me?" The worst part for Michele was that she knew about Dr. Clark's recommendations before this happened. We have a hard time believing things we can't see, which is why Michele wanted me to include her heartbreaking story here. Now she pays close attention to even the small things such as Styrofoam containers.

Don't drink from Styrofoam cups. Styrene is toxic. Avoid foods packaged in aluminum. Avoid using aluminum foil. If you must use it, be sure the foil doesn't touch the food. The hazards of the metal we consume daily in our food, beverages and products we use on our bodies are well documented. I prefer to get my essential minerals from food, not from toxic items. This conversion was really very easy and I believe the benefits of safe cooking go a long way when it comes to dealing with cancer.

When it comes to the kitchen, there are plenty of habits that you can improve. For example, I have several cutting boards in my kitchen. One is specifically for meat. I NEVER use the same cutting board for vegetables and fruits as I use for meat! Anyone who has ever been in my kitchen knows which cutting board is for meat only! I feel very strongly about this and there is never an exception to this rule in my kitchen.

Some other good tips for the kitchen include keeping the counters, sinks and tables clean. You can do this by wiping them down with grain alcohol. Grain alcohol does not contain chemicals or other solvents often found in commercial cleaners. If you have a problem with ants, use vinegar on your wiping cloth. It leaves a residue that keeps ants away. Vinegar is a safe way to keep ants away from the outside of your house, too. You can pour vinegar all around the outside of your home. Use about one gallon for every five feet. Doing this several times a year is a lot safer than using commercial poisons.

I separate my sponges – one for dishes and one for the counter and tabletops. Throw them away and replace them with new sponges frequently. Also, make sure to dry them out completely each day. After you use a sponge, it absorbs all sorts of yucky bacteria. Of course, after you use it, the last thing you do is wring it out, transferring all that bacteria to your hands!

Some people use rubber gloves for cleaning the kitchen. This is probably a very good idea. But if you're like most people, you probably don't use rubber gloves; so wash your hands carefully after squeezing out that sponge.

The same is true for your kitchen towels. I change out the towels for fresh ones often. I seem to go through a lot of paper towels, too. I don't like this because of the environmental impact, but sometimes I can't avoid it for sanitation purposes. This is why I have lots of kitchen towels and I pay close attention to how I use them. If I'm drying the table or counter with a towel, I don't use it for the dishes or drying my hands. I know this may seem a little extreme, but I prefer to err on the safe side.

Rinsing your hands with grain alcohol is a good way to keep them sanitized. Sanitized or not, never put your fingers in your mouth. This includes biting your fingernails. Think about the amount of germs and bacteria on your hands – particularly under your fingernails. Follow these sanitation rules at all times, not just when you're in the kitchen. And teach your children to do the same.

When preparing meat, pork, poultry or fish, I try to never touch it with my bare hands. As you know, I don't normally eat any type of meat, but I do prepare it for my husband, family and guests. I don't expect everyone to conform to my eating habits, so I have no issues with what others eat. When I clean and prepare these things, I use plastic gloves or a meat fork to keep anything from coming in contact with my skin. You may think this is a bit extreme, but it's just a habit I've picked up after cancer.

Many of my new habits revolve around the kitchen. I eat as much organic food as possible mainly because it contains much less dye and pesticide pollution than conventionally grown foods.

Kosher foods are also very healthy. Dr. Clark made an interesting discovery about kosher food. She found that most food labeled "kosher" contain no asbestos, azo dye, lanthanide, heavy metal, acrylic acid or urethane. She discovered that kosher food didn't even have rabbit fluke! So when you shop, put kosher and organic at the top of your list.

I've learned a lot about food and the importance of a clean kitchen. It's not just a matter of keeping your kitchen clean – properly cleaning your food is crucial. Dr. Clark's theory on parasites has me cleaning my food in an entirely new way. There are more than parasites on food. Dr. Clark has also found asbestos, dye and lanthanide on food. You may wonder how asbestos can get on your food. It's likely that the food picks it up from conveyor belts that contain asbestos.

I used to think that washing my food and scrubbing it well under running water was sufficient. Unfortunately, it's not possible to wash off parasites this way. Many people think using a commercial produce wash is better, but Dr. Clark found that these cleaners contain solvents and isopropyl alcohol. So instead of cleaning your food, you have now added one of the key toxins all cancer patients must avoid – isopropyl alcohol. The good news is that you can rid your food of these toxins and parasites by following a simple process. Here's what I do:

1. Soak all greens, vegetables and fruit in a solution of water and five percent (5%) hydrochloric acid to remove parasites. I use two drops of five percent (5%) hydrochloric acid per one cup of water. Soak for one minute, no longer. If you soak longer, parasites will re-enter the food. I then rinse, dry and store the food. You can also clean parasites off with a rinse of Lugol's iodine, one drop per quart of water. I stay away from this method in case someone is allergic to iodine. I prefer to use the hydrochloric acid method.

2. If the food has dye or benzene (pesticide) contamination you can add vitamin B2 powder to the hydrochloric acid wash. Only a pinch is needed.

3. I use a hot water soak for avocados and bananas to remove any spray wax, asbestos, dye, lanthanide and benzene. I soak them twice in hot water for one minute each time, drying both times.

4. Wash eggs thoroughly and dry with a paper towel. Never put the eggs back in the carton. The carton is full of salmonella. Dr. Clark has never found salmonella inside eggs, only on the outer shell. She believes the salmonella found in eggs happens when the un-cleaned eggshell is cracked, transferring the salmonella into the egg.

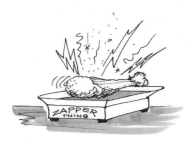

My favorite way of removing parasites from foods is by zapping them. I purchased a special plate called a zappicator, that I can set my food on and actually zap the parasites off it. The zapper is a device invented by Dr. Clark. She describes a zapper as any unit that generates a positive offset square wave frequency between 10 Hz and 500,000 Hz using a nine-volt battery. The food zappicator contains an electro-magnet attached to a zapper. This changes the food's polarization to north. The food is actually fresher then. The zappicator can destroy viruses, bacteria, parasites and do much more than this brief description. You can read more about zappers and the food zappicator in Dr. Clark's book, *The Cure for HIV and AIDS*.

I simply place the food on the zapper plate for seven minutes. If the item contains cheese, dairy or eggs, I zap it for an additional seven minutes. It's that simple. This is an easy method for killing parasites at all stages, even their eggs. Because the depth of the food isn't an issue, even meat, poultry, pork, fish and nuts can be cleaned. Once the food has been zapped, it is parasite-free. "Zapping" doesn't affect the vitamins and nutrients or change the food in any noticeable way other than to rid it of parasites. This is one of the best investments I've made when it comes to eating healthy. You can find food zappicators on the Internet. I also have other zappers for personal use.

I have a couple different types of zappers that I use to zap myself. The first one was homemade, very inexpensive, easy to use and effective. Dr. Clark really enjoyed seeing my handmade version. She gives instructions on making these zappers in her books. I also have what's called a plate zapper. With this zapper, you can target specific organs, zapping them individually. I realize this sounds rather mysterious, but once you learn about the benefits of zapping, it's really very simple. You can find lots of information about Dr. Clark and her zappers on the Internet and in her books.

I truly believe the change in my kitchen habits has been one of the most rewarding improvements in my life. I'm proud to have dinner guests and I'm confident that the food they eat in my home is healthy and nourishing. Trust me, these changes will make the time you spend in your kitchen more enjoyable and rewarding than you can imagine. It is gratifying to know the food you prepare is clean, safe and genuinely life-giving.

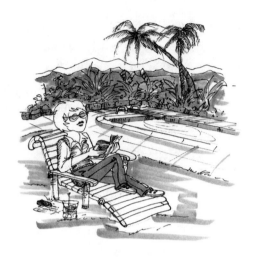

Get Out

Get out of the house whenever possible. You don't even have to go anywhere. You can simply sit outside. When I was going through chemo or just feeling like something on the bottom of a shoe, I'd sit in my back yard. I'd sit in the sun and feel its warmth. I'm not saying to go out and abuse yourself in the sun. I'm saying to spend some healthy time outdoors. Every living thing needs fresh air and sunshine.

Ever notice how cats and dogs lounge in the sun? Do they know something we don't? We all need the sun to stay healthy. It provides us with vitamin D and helps us metabolize other vitamins in our bodies. The sun provides many benefits, so don't hide from it. You should get at least twenty minutes of sunshine every day. It's not just about sunshine – it's about fresh air, too.

There is a lot of information about how things in our homes contribute to our illnesses. There's paint, fabrics, chemical cleaners and all sorts of other manmade items in our homes. All these products emit something that eventually ends up in our lungs. Open up your windows and allow fresh air in whenever possible. If you're sick with any type of serious illness, I suggest you do a home clean-up, just as you did with your kitchen.

Once you learn about the products in your home and how they can affect your health, you'll wonder why you hadn't thought about this before now. And if you think these items don't have an impact on your well-being, ask anyone who's had to deal with a moldy home. Asthma patients are often told to replace carpeting with hardwood floors or tile. Many things in your home may slow down your recovery. Home clean-up is an easy task because it mostly involves getting rid of things or relocating them to a safe place, such as a detached garage.

Get rid of all chemical cleaners. You shouldn't store or use these items in your home. They are toxins and they don't help in your recovery. If your garage is attached to your home, you'll need to clean that up, too. Fumes from the many chemicals stored there can easily seep into your home, especially if you enter your home through the garage. I absolutely suggest learning more about this topic.

Remember, we are trying to give our poor immune systems a break. It's all these little things that add up to big results. And even after you do your home clean-up, don't forget to spend plenty of time outside.

Getting out of the house helps you both mentally and physically. The more time you spend outdoors, the better you will feel. If you don't have a yard, then sit on your porch or go out to your apartment courtyard. I found that life was different in my back yard than it was inside my home. Yes, I was still sick when I was outside, but I didn't have the same mental perspective as when I was in bed or on the couch watching television. In the back yard I watched the clouds, the birds, even the wind in the trees.

Get a birdbath or a fountain. I am lucky enough to have a fountain in the yard that draws in lots of birds. It's amazing how many types of birds visit my yard. I often recognize seasonal birds, just passing through. Other birds are regulars and are there daily. Another thing I noticed was that certain birds visit at certain times of the day. I became so interested that I actually bought a book about identifying birds. I learned the names of the many types of birds in my neighborhood. I had lived here for years and had never taken time to notice all the activity in my own yard. It took cancer to get me to sit still long enough to notice.

Mostly I sat in the shade of my patio. I used binoculars to get close-up details of the birds. The birds alone caused me to want to spend more time outside. I looked forward to seeing "who" would visit the fountain each day. Once you start, you'll notice all sorts of things in your yard. There are butterflies that float, squirrels that tease the dog, lizards that sunbathe, bunnies that munch the grass and more. Rabbits came very early in the morning or at dusk. I was astounded by all the wildlife that resides here in the city and you will be, too, no matter where you live. The best part is that you can sit in your back yard without worrying about how you look or what you wear. Simply relax, enjoy the sunshine, breathe in the fresh air and let nature assist you in your healing. It's just so very good to get out of the house.

My back yard was my retreat, especially during that first six months. With all my physical issues, chemo and the colostomy, I simply didn't feel like doing much. I'll admit there were times when I went out and socialized. I even went with my husband to his twenty-year class reunion. These outings took great preparation and mental strength, but the rewards were tremendous. I could visualize myself as healthy again and I looked forward to the future.

The point I'm trying to make is that even if you can only drag your ragged battered self out to the yard, plop down in a chair and do nothing, you will feel better. When you are in your yard watching the sky or anything else, it takes your focus off of your illness. It keeps you in the present moment. Stress comes from resisting the present moment. No matter how uncomfortable the current situation may be, you can eliminate the stress associated with it by acknowledging and accepting it for what it is. This will bring you back to the present moment and the present is where healing occurs.

When you are in the house and you are sick, there's a tendency to dwell on your symptoms. Inside the house, you do things like get on the Internet to read more about your illness, its side effects and other problematic issues. You watch television to see if Montel is going to be talking about miracle cures. The house seems to take on an air of illness. Going outside exposes you to new light, new sounds and new smells. The more you focus on things that are pleasant, the better you will feel. You don't need to do anything, just sit there and find pleasure outside. Even if it's raining, you can bundle up and sit on the patio. Being out of the house is what's important. You'll find it calming and peaceful.

There is balance in nature and there is healing. Allow the earth and nature to capture your attention. After all, you are part of this great universe; don't underestimate your importance here. You are part of this balance. Nature will assist you in reclaiming your health and well-being.

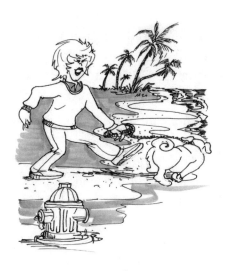

Adventures in the Hood

I decided to take up walking, wondering just how far I could go. I felt hot wearing my wig and I felt so darned weak. I had to wear the wig, though. I didn't want to go outside looking like something that would frighten small children. Without my wig, I wasn't just bald; I had no eyebrows and no eyelashes. I looked thin and frail. My outer shell reflected the war within. Perhaps it was my dread of strangers gawking at me or maybe I felt my own vulnerability. Whatever it was, I just wanted to be normal again, even if it was only for a short time. I needed to walk anonymously.

I had to start getting some of my strength back and walking was the only form of exercise I could manage. I probably benefited more mentally from the walk than I did physically. I returned home feeling victorious after completing a small but strenuous lap around the entire block. At that moment, I was actually happy. Although it was a small thing, I felt it was a new beginning. Walking turned out to be something I looked forward to each day. It surprised me how the time I spent walking not only strengthened my body but also strengthened my mind and fed my spirit.

When I was alone at home, I was comfortable and preferred a hat or scarf instead of a hot itchy wig. So, one of those days I went to the curb to retrieve the mail. Usually my timing was good and I got the mail without being noticed, but not that day. On that day, my neighbor Shirley spotted me in "the hat that did little to hide my baldness." I barely knew Shirley, but in the blink of an eye, there she was, standing beside me, concerned and supportive. Our short conversation left me feeling warm and uplifted. I never expected such kindness from a near stranger, neighbor or not. It wasn't as though she lived next door. No, she lived all the way down the street. Shirley turned out to be one of those people who is simply a pleasure to be around. She has a special energy that makes others feel good. I wish I could say her response to my baldness resulted in me being able to let go of my wigs and concealing cosmetics in public, but that just didn't happen. However, it did help me relax about reactions from my neighbors.

Soon I met more neighbors. A simple hello often led to an introduction that later led to more conversation. While I continued to walk wearing my mask of wigs and cosmetics, I got to know my neighborhood and its unique social characteristics.

No matter where you go, each neighborhood seems to have a personality of its own. For example, the people in my "hood" actually make an effort to meet each other. The families who live here organize block parties. They include bounce houses or water slides, piñatas and other activities for the kids. We have the street closed off for safety and everyone brings food. We meet newcomers and long-time homeowners. Meeting the families, their children and learning who lives where creates a real sense of community. Even though I was ill, I made sure to attend our block parties. I already knew several neighbors and looked forward to meeting more.

My regular walks increased my visibility in the neighborhood. I met lots of people through my walks. I learned that I wasn't the only one who held the cancer card. That attractive widow, Bert, always active, walking or working in her yard, also held the card. I wouldn't have known it because she takes care of herself and has a wonderful outlook on life. She has battled cancer off and on throughout her life and recently finished another round of chemo. There are others. While the type of cancer varies, the pain and the suffering that comes with treatment is much the same.

Finding a cancer community right here in my small neighborhood opened my eyes a little more. We exchange stories and phone numbers and provide each other with support and encouragement. It's very comforting to know your neighbors are close by and willing to help. It's often easier than calling a family member who is some distance away or perhaps busy. I never guessed that I would gain so much from something as simple as walking regularly in my own neighborhood.

Over the years, I've reclaimed my health and vitality and I've joyously returned to favorite physical activities such as tennis and more. While these activities consume much of my time, they haven't replaced my regular walks in the hood. There is real value in connecting with your neighbors.

The essence, energy and the feel of a neighborhood reflect the wonderful souls who live there. My walks have become a routine that's as regular to me as any habit. When I feel like slacking off, I use my dog, Buzz, as a motivator. After all, he must be walked!

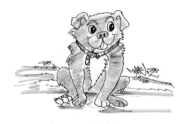

The best part of this is the fun I've discovered in walking. At first, I dreaded it when the weather was bad; cold winds, pounding rain and summer heat waves made me want to stay inside. But I walked through it all. In the summer, I walked early in the morning or even waited until dark. Summer nights can be unbelievably beautiful. Walking under the stars, seeing the moon rise, even night clouds can turn a simple walk into something quite spiritual. I even found a spot where I can view the city lights. It's not always so pleasant, though! I've walked during nights when it's overcast and so dark that I can't see a thing. That's when other things come into focus. The way homes look at night is different. Yards are transformed with lighting and homes change with holiday or party decorations. I compare dark silent houses with the lively noisy lighted ones. Sounds and smells waft from homes. The aroma of home cooking and the sounds of a practicing drummer are only some of the things that come to mind. There are always other walkers (often with dogs), sometimes bicyclists, skateboarders or someone with a baby in a stroller. It seems like once the summer sun goes down, the neighborhood comes to life.

The winter months are a different story, especially if it is raining or blowing cold wind. I look at these walks as an adventure. Bundling up in rain gear, ski clothes or whatever is appropriate, I venture out. The first time I did this, I wondered how long it had been since I had played in the rain. I've been all grown up for too long. We grown-ups have a tendency to avoid this type of stuff. Here I was, feeling exhilarated and alive again. Now I delight in the changes. The skyline looks different with leafless trees. Summer flowers give way to sturdier winter plants. Sometimes the sky puts on a full-blown show, with color-ful cloud formations racing, dancing and moving along. Animals are always a bonus on walks. Some birds sing to you, some perch willingly or curiously while others display their beauty in flight. There is so much to appreciate and walking gives me time to contemplate it. I refer to these daily jaunts as my spiritual walks.

I use this time to think about all sorts of things and to nur-ture myself with positive affirmations. I say things to myself such as, "I'm healthy and beautiful. I am loving and kind." I think things such as this until I get to the point where I feel myself in that place where it's no longer just words. I actu-ally feel healthy. I feel beautiful, kind and loving and it feels so good. Sometimes I think about goals I've set; then I focus on that indescribable feeling of achieving those goals. Some of my goals are material in nature, but most are not. The times I've experienced my greatest joys usually have noth-ing to do with material objects. Often my goals are along the lines of, "I want people to feel good, secure and comfortable around me. I want the children in my life to know they are safe and deeply loved. I want others to see how beautiful and magnificent they truly are." These goals may sound way out there to you, but your priorities tend to change in a big way when you are standing at death's doorstep.

Believe me; I still say positive affirmations that apply to money and all the modern-day comforts of life. It just depends on where my head is that day. My material affirmations get as much attention as the others. I playfully work with my visualizations and words until I reach the point of attaining the excitement and joy that accompany them. Words and visualizations mean little without the emotion behind them. So when I'm not socializing with neighbors, I use my walking time to improve my spiritual self as well as my physical self.

Now, you don't get all this from one or two walks around the block. It took months before I started getting to know people and tuning into the details of my neighborhood. For me, walking is part of my healing routine because it involves the physical, the mental and the spiritual. I've been walking in my neighborhood for years now and, believe it or not, new people and discoveries still pop up.

Just recently, I took Buzz on a long walk. It was a hot day, but I felt like getting out anyway. I took a couple of poop bags, some ice water and off we went. Buzz is quite a character. He's a small dog, a Pug-Pekinese mix. Some people think he's ugly, with his under-bite and crooked nose. But most people see past these flaws because of his obedience, obvious desire to please and his spunky personality. Buzz is always excited and happy. He loves his walks in any weather; particularly the long walks. But long walks do take a toll on little Buzz and when they do, he lets you know immediately. He finds a lush spot on the curbside grass and just stops dead in his tracks. He sprawls out like a bear skin rug, with his front and back legs stretched out as far as they'll go. At this point, there's no moving him. You can pull, tug or even drag him, but nothing works. Buzz is going to take a break and that's that! I am left to sit crossed-legged waiting patiently for who knows how long.

It was on one of these breaks, close to home, that I met George. As his car slowed to get a closer look at the little dog sprawled out on the grass, he stopped. I 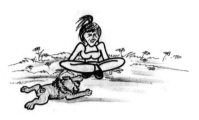 heard his laughter and he said, "I wish I had a camera!" He continued with cheerful comments such as how we'd all like to sprawl out like that in the heat and we moved to introductions. George has been in the neighborhood a long time. He lives a couple of blocks from me on a dead-end street. Perhaps that's why we hadn't met until that day.

When George asked me what I did for a living, it caught me off guard. I was hesitant and even felt a little squeamish. The quick and confident response I'd been accustomed to giving all my life was no longer valid. My career days had ended years ago with the arrival of ovarian cancer. I wasn't out there in the corporate world any more, but I was working on this book every day, so that was my job. I took a deep breath and summoned up the courage to say out loud, "I'm writing a book."

George's next question made me even more uncomfortable, but it was only logical for him to ask, "What's the book about?" What had I been thinking? Why hadn't I just told him that I was retired or temporarily unemployed? I wasn't really comfortable with revealing this type of personal information to a complete stranger, but I had no choice. I sucked it up and told him the book was about my battles with ovarian cancer. I didn't know how he would react. My nervous feelings came to an abrupt end as George revealed his own story of survival.

By George's description, he should be dead. He is here against all odds and despite conventional medicine. His prostate cancer was so advanced and severe that surgery was not even an option. His doctors told him that he could take some drugs that might keep him around for a year or so, but there was nothing more they could do.

George searched for a cure for months. He sought out top physicians and consulted with all sorts of experts in the field. His search took him to Mexico and Texas – anywhere he could find hope. Doctor after doctor confirmed the grim diagnosis. He used four months of precious time tirelessly searching, only to end up exactly where he had started. He finally accepted his fate. It seemed there was only one place left to turn, so George turned to God.

George's story is fascinating because it is a story of miracles. Not many people believe in miracles these days, but a miracle happened to George. His was not a desperate last-ditch attempt to bargain with a God that George had neglected and forgotten long ago. No, George had always believed in God. While he certainly isn't a fanatic about it, he'd kept up with his faith and attended church regularly. So when Sunday rolled around, it wasn't unusual that George went to church and prayed. His were not the routine prayers of one who regularly attends church. George's prayers that day were the deep emotional prayers of one who is dying.

During his prayers that day, George saw a pinprick of light. As he focused on the light, it grew brighter. As the light continued to brighten, it started to grow. It grew larger and larger until he was completely engulfed by the light. Kneeling there in church, shaking as tears streamed down his cheeks, George clearly heard the words, "I am with you and you will be fine."

Realizing he was still in church, George looked around and was stunned to see that no one had even noticed what had just taken place. No one had noticed the event, no one had seen that he was shaking – not even his tear-stained face brought the slightest bit of attention. George quickly approached the Monsignor and exclaimed, "God was here and there was a miracle in this church!" The Monsignor's reply seemed almost nonchalant. He said something along the lines of, "Yes, I know. God is always here."

"No, no, you don't understand," George insisted. Unable to contain his joy, George tried to explain his experience and the miracle that had happened to him. The Monsignor calmly asked him hold the discussion until services ended. That left George alone to contemplate the miracle and his next steps.

The next day, George went to his doctor and demanded surgery. He stressed that he had insurance, he had money and he had a miracle! He wouldn't accept no for an answer. Somehow, he was able to convince his doctor to operate and immediately began the pre-op requirements.

After the operation, his surgeon came into the recovery room to discuss the outcome. Her befuddled look instantly raised George's curiosity. She explained that her findings in surgery weren't what she'd expected at all. She said his prostate had a hole in it, where she could only assume the cancer had somehow escaped into his body. The tissue she saw was not the unhealthy tissue of disease; rather it looked like the pink and fresh new tissue of a baby. She was certain his body was still riddled with cancer and the pathology reports that would validate it would be ready in the morning.

Very early the following day, the door flew open. Instead of his surgeon, twenty-two doctors filled the room, surrounding his bed. George, a bit astounded by the early-morning parade, asked, "Does it take twenty-two doctors to read a pathology report?" His doctor's reply was the best thing imaginable, "All these doctors are here to see what a miracle looks like."

Now I know what a miracle looks like, too. It looks like my neighbor George!

If I hadn't been walking in my neighborhood regularly, I would never have heard George's story. To think that I could discover a miracle anywhere – let alone in my own neighborhood – was something I'd never even considered. Until I met George, I'd never known anyone who had a miracle healing. I think it's valuable to include his story here because it emphasizes the amazing healing possibilities that are all around us. Miracles can – and do – happen.

Even though George had a miracle healing, he doesn't take it for granted. In fact, George introduced me to one of my favorite products, Immunocal. George swears by Immunocal and its ability to enhance the immune system. You don't have to have a prescription to buy Immunocal, but it is included in the "Physician's Desk Reference," used by doctors and health professionals for prescribing medication, dosage and additional information on medication. Immunocal, a natural food protein concentrate, is made under strict conditions to maintain its integrity. You can easily obtain this product and information about it by searching the key word

"Immunocal" on the Internet. Learning about Immunocal is another benefit I gained by walking in my neighborhood.

It's true that not all neighborhoods are like mine. You may think that your neighborhood won't have treasures like mine does because you live in an apartment, or on a busy street or near a college. Or perhaps the thought of a block party in your neighborhood seems absurd. Don't let your preconceived notions stop you. You'll find that life's treasures are everywhere. You can find lots of things by taking walks. You don't have to leave town or go someplace else to have an inspiring experience. You can get healthier, meet people, feed your spirit and enjoy nature (sky, birds and plants are all around you) simply by opening your front door and stepping out. Even something as simple as a stroll around the block can turn into an adventure in the "hood."

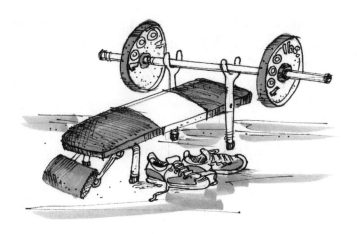

Exercise

Here's a subject I think many of us would like to ignore, especially when dealing with cancer. Even before cancer, I was never good about going to the gym or working out on a regular basis. Sure, I'd joined a local health club plenty of times with the very best of intentions, but I never stuck with it. My idea of exercise was usually an outdoor activity such as swimming, tennis or hiking. I enjoyed these activities and participated in them regularly. But ovarian cancer quickly put a quick stop to that.

After my initial surgery, I wasn't able to do much of anything. My chemotherapy started before I'd even had a chance to recover from the extreme operation. Side effects from the Taxol and Carboplatin were far worse than I'd ever imagined. I also had a rough time managing and coping with the temporary colostomy. I was just a wreck. The best I could do during the first six months was to get dressed and attempt to look as good as possible. Exercise was out of the question. I could barely function. Usually, I just sat in my back yard and watched the birds as I counted the days until my next surgery and having my colostomy reversed.

After my second-look surgery in July, I started to see the light at the end of the proverbial tunnel! I was no longer plagued with the colostomy, but I saw that it would be a while before I would be able to resume a normal routine. My body needed time to adjust and that meant staying close to the toilet. I was still bald and wearing a wig; it would take a while for hair growth. So I spent the next couple of months recuperating.

Although I looked forward to getting back into shape, by October, I had started having issues with the Panacryl. Once the Panacryl began worming its way out of my abdomen, it was endless pain. Pulling the Panacryl suture material out of my incision scar became a full-time job. Just the thought of exercise was a joke. I could barely stand up straight. I always had open wounds that needed to be packed. This ritual consumed the remainder of 2000 and all of 2001. I prayed the New Year would signal the end of my Panacryl ordeal. Thankfully, it did.

I began to walk and play tennis again. I was in horrible condition, but I had fun again. For the first time in years, I could move my body and it felt very good. I just couldn't get enough of it. I signed up for a tennis class and met new people. I finally started to feel strength in my muscles. I was coming back to life, but by April, the cancer had already returned. I'd enjoyed a few months of normality, but then it was gone – just like that!

I can't explain the dread that overwhelmed me. I knew I wasn't physically strong enough to go through cancer again, but then what choice did I have? I had a third operation and another series of chemo. In May 2003, I endured my last chemo treatment. In total, more than three years had passed and I was back where I'd started, yet not quite. Things were different. Physically, I was like a marshmallow. Mentally, I was teetering. I had propped myself up for so many years, but I no longer had that firm conviction of being able to beat cancer. I knew all too well that once ovarian cancer returns, you might as well just sign off, because it's over. My hopes of being in that small percentage of survivors ended when the cancer returned. I knew how quickly women went once recurrences started. I'd seen it over and over with other ovarian cancer patients. I felt as though I was empty shell, operating on remote and just trying to come to terms with death. I felt lonely and insecure, but I kept my feelings to myself because I didn't want to be more of a burden than I already was. Privately, I was exhausted and depleted, but publicly I stuck to my routines and made time for family and friends.

In December 2003, Dolby and I went out for lunch. As usual, she looked fabulous. Dolby has a great figure and spares no expense on looking good. On that day, like most others, she was simply radiant. She was the picture of health and I was the picture of death. I remember looking at her, longing for that genuine feeling she radiated. I told her, "I only wish I could look as good as you do." Her response was, "Are you kidding? You sure can, girl. Don't you belong to a gym?" For once, I responded honestly, "No, what's the use? I'm dying." I'll never forget her reply. She said, "Honey, we're all dying."

She was right. We are all dying. Why not feel as good as possible in the meantime? I kept asking myself, "What will it take to get that healthy glow of beauty back?" I knew that every muscle in my body was weak and needed work, but I couldn't see myself joining a health club. Physically, I felt incapable of determining what would be a safe and healthy workout for me, considering my current state and everything I had been through. I bluntly faced myself and demanded answers. Well, the answer came the next day.

I remembered a small gym in the shopping center where I did my marketing. I decided to drive over and check it out. It was called L.A. Private Trainers. I liked the name and the location was perfect. So I went in to investigate. My first impression was relief. It wasn't one of those commercial places that required tour guides and had models and hunks filling every room. Usually I feel somewhat intimidated when I go into a gym, but not here. L.A. Private Trainers had a more intimate feel to it. It felt like a place for locals. I saw people getting help on an individual basis, which was exactly what I needed. After getting all the details, prices and options, I decided to sign up.

Given my situation, I decided to meet with a personal trainer three days a week. My first appointment was devoted to evaluating the state of my health at that time. The trainer took my body weight and measurements. The first visit included assessments of everything, including my health history and my physical abilities and limitations. I learned that my physical abilities on everything, from flexibility to strength, were in the "poor to fair" category. I had a long way to go, but I'd taken the first and most critical step. I was there! I worked out with a personal trainer every Monday,

Wednesday and Friday. I met other people in the gym and saw them overcoming their physical and health challenges, too. It wasn't just about looking good; it was about being healthy and strong.

The trainers were amazing. They were compassionate and supportive. They shared in every victory and motivated me in the most sincere way. I grew stronger, both physically and mentally. Working out impacted me in more ways than I expected. I regained my self-confidence and, most importantly, my self-esteem. I was happier and felt proud of my accomplishments. The constant stress I was under about my recurring illness and weakened condition seemed to disintegrate. Stress is a major contributor to all types of illness, so this may have been the most vital benefit of all. I no longer dwelled on death; instead I concentrated on my new physical goals. The stronger I got, the healthier my outlook became.

I even took advantage of the dietician on staff. She taught me about the glycemic index and how I could use it to improve my health. She also measured my metabolic rate to determine how many calories I should consume each day. We went over diet recommendations and made adjustments according to my particular desires. For example, I prefer to eat only organic and non-processed food, so we replaced many of the low calorie pre-packaged snacks on the lists with fresh fruit or vegetables. We also made adjustments around meat and chicken since I avoid that almost entirely. I learned I could eat a variety of healthy food without worrying about a lack of nutrition.

L.A. Private Trainers played a crucial role in my recovery. I knew if I were ever going to stick with a workout routine, I would need help and personal attention. If someone was there waiting for me, I'd be there. That was my reality. If that's what it takes for you to work out, then just admit it and go from there. When I started, I wasn't sure I would stick with it, but I did. From December 2003 to February 2005, I worked out faithfully three times a week with a personal trainer. It was awesome and the results exceeded my expectations.

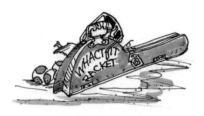

You may not need a gym or a personal trainer like I did, but you do need to work out regularly. If you are one of those people who can pop in a video and follow along at home, then go for it! If you have a bike, then ride it. If you can walk, then walk in your neighborhood. Whatever you can do to get exercise, do it! Nothing makes you feel as good as when your body starts to get stronger and you truly start to feel healthier. You must make exercise a regular part of your new life; there's no way around it. If you are feeling low, discouraged – or even defeated as I felt, exercise will change all that. Give it a try. I'm sure you will be as surprised as I was to learn that exercise heals your mind, body and spirit.

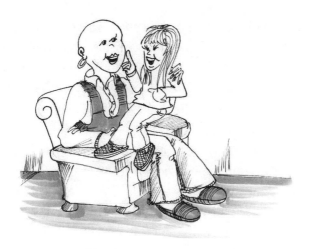

Baby Love

Oh, nothing compares to baby love! I was fortunate enough to have babies around me during all my cancer illnesses and treatments. It doesn't matter if they are nieces, nephews, grandchildren or any children, they can really give healing. It's not just the love you give to them; it's the love they give back to you. Children are the personification of unconditional love. Is there anything healthier than that?

I remember one evening when my grandson Mason spent the night with us. He was so cute and precious. He went to sleep in his crib, but later in the night he woke up. I was so tired from chemo that I put him in bed with Grandpa and me. Since we had a king-size bed, there was plenty of room. I, in my cute little nightcap, fell back to sleep without much thought. When I awoke, the nightcap was gone and there I was as bald as could be. Mason had never seen me without hair and I was afraid I was going to scare the poor little boy to death. He took one look at me, and with great surprise in his eyes, he squealed, "Grandma, I love you." Then he threw his arms around me and bounced with joy to find himself in Grandma and Grandpa's bed. I'll never forget that morning. Mason never even noticed I was bald. Now that's some kind of love!

There was also the day my sister Cathy came to visit and brought my loving niece, Roxanne. As we sat on the patio, discussing my upcoming second-look surgery and the end of chemo, I mentioned how I was looking forward to having hair again, especially eyelashes. She asked when my eyelashes would come back and I told her, "Very soon, because I am all done with my treatments." Roxanne was sitting on my lap, looking up at me very intently. She excitedly said, "Look Auntie Chris, it's happening, you have one eyelash!" Well, leave it to a child to spot one eyelash. Guess what? After she left, I looked for that eyelash. Yes, things were looking up. I did indeed have one eyelash! You take your joy wherever you can find it.

One time, we watched Mason for a week while my daughter and son-in-law were on vacation. I guess Mason was about three years old then. I asked his parents if I could take him to the movies since he hadn't been to a real theater yet. Up to then, we had only watched videos. You know how kids are. I had to sit through *Jungle Book* about fifty times, including all the previews. Heaven forbid we should skip the previews! We wouldn't want to miss the endless advertising of "movies coming soon to theaters near you."

Anyway, his parents agreed that we could go to a real movie theater, so we went to a matinee to see *Finding Nemo*. It was so much fun. We had popcorn and lemonade while we watched the movie. At one point, Mason jumped up and announced – very loudly, "Grandma, I have to go potty. Let's run!" Well, of course the entire audience burst out laughing as we ran out of the theater. Of course, we had to run back so we wouldn't miss anything. We had a blast that day and went home when the movie was over.

Mason couldn't wait for Grandpa to come home from work. He wanted to tell him all about "Finding Nemo." Sure enough, when Grandpa stepped through the door, Mason ran up to him squealing, "Grandpa, Grandpa! Guess what? Grandma took me to the real coming to theaters near you soon!" Needless to say, Les and I laughed about that for days. I am just crazy about all the children in my family.

During illness and during health, the children have been a great gift to me. I adore the feeling when my tiny grandson Vincent clings to me and won't let go. I love the way he taps my chest and in his baby talk, smiles and says, "Grandma." I am lucky to be able to pick up Mason and Vincent from school, take them to my home and spend time with them. It's a lot of work, but it's work I love. When I see the importance of my role as a grandmother and aunt, I realize my value in this world. My sister Cathy gave me a photo of my niece with a saying on the frame that reads:

One hundred years from now, it will not matter
what kind of car I drove or what kind of clothes I wore.
All that will matter is that I made a difference
in the life of a child.

I could go on and on with stories about each of my grandchildren, nieces and nephews. Each one is precious and loving. I am incredibly proud of these children and their accomplishments. Just watching them grow and being part of their lives is a gift. Children are the joyous expression of an untainted life. They are truly in the moment and grounded to the here and now. I could tell you about how each of them individually contributed to my healing and my joy, but that would take another book.

Although I see some of the children in my family more than others, due to distance and work schedules, I adore each of them. I am very lucky and I feel blessed to have been able to develop such special bonds. Children are natural healers. Open your arms and let them in with all their innocence, beauty, truth and unconditional love.

I've read that children laugh more than 300 times a day and adults laugh maybe 15 times a day. No wonder we're sick! Spend a day with children. They will get you laughing. It's impossible to feel stress with so much love and fun going on. All that laughing will lift your spirits and the best part is that you'll laugh yourself to improved health. Love and laughter is a beautiful combination, don't you agree? Having the love of a child nurtures the adult as much as it does the child. A child's love is pure and powerful. If you have children around you, embrace them; their value is undeniable.

Each of us is valuable in countless ways. Remember your worth. You are here for a purpose, whether you recognize that purpose or not. Please don't leave us prematurely. We need you and your love, especially the children around you. Children can never get too much love and they are responsive to your love and attention. Healing comes in many forms and children can be joyous contributors. Embrace your children and embrace your health.

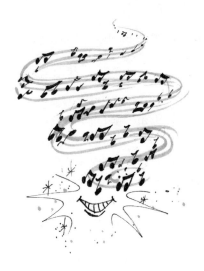

Music

Music is a wonderful way to raise your vibration. Raising your vibration is about raising your frequency. Everything in the universe is made of energy and each form vibrates at a different speed. When you resonate at a higher frequency, you increase your awareness and open yourself to new possibilities that previously may have seemed impossible. There are numerous ways to raise your vibration. I have mentioned many in this book, such as affirmations of gratitude, love, joy and peace. Visualization, journaling and forgiveness also raise your vibration. You might try meditation, yoga or Tai Chi. Anything that is positive and creates a good feeling can raise your vibration.

When you play beautiful music, you feel its effects immediately. Have you noticed how music can change your mood? It can take you to your grandest or saddest moments.

When you think of music in its simplest terms, you think about how it makes you feel.

Just the other day, I saw a car full of teenage girls singing at the top of their lungs. Even though they weren't great singers, they were smiling, bouncing and clapping their hands while proudly singing out of the car's open windows. I couldn't help but smile along with them. Just witnessing this joyous moment raised my vibration. They sang directly to me. I found myself laughing and grinning back at them, sharing in their joy. I just couldn't stop myself.

Oh sure, the little voice in the back of my mind worried about teenage drivers and their distractions from the road, but I squashed that thought. Since my worrying couldn't accomplish anything, I purposely took that negative thought and reworded it into a positive one. I said, "After that song, I'll bet the driver tones them all down for safety." Then I went back to embracing the moment. I realized then that music really does affect us on a cellular level.

You usually select music that makes you feel a certain way. Music can make you feel any emotion. Sometimes, your favorite music is exhilarating and at other times, it seems you're just not into that particular music at all. I think the music you select is the closest to your current mood, which indicates your current vibration level. It seems you can't simply jump to a vibration that's too far from your current situation. In other words, when you're feeling sick or when you're in pain, you're probably not in the mood to blast rock and roll music.

When I felt miserable, I listened to healing music. I tried to find any type of music labeled as healing. These choices always seemed to make me feel better. I've heard women say that they listened to classical music during pregnancy to benefit their unborn children. I also recall experiments with plants. People have recorded how plants reacted to a variety of music. Masaru Emoto documented how water molecules responded to various types of music. It seems that beautiful music always produces beautiful results. It doesn't matter if it is unborn children, plants or water – all respond to music. For these reasons, I listened to healing music when I felt lousy. I'll admit, though, there were times when I didn't make the healing music choice.

Being human, there were times when I purposely indulged in sad or heart-wrenching music, knowing death was standing over me. I thought about dedicating certain songs to my husband, family or friends at my funeral. I know it sounds pathetic, but it helped me in a way. I felt depressed, so why not let it out through music? I found there was plenty of music to echo my misery. Wallowing in self-pity isn't exactly healthy, but it sure helped me in the moment. To put it bluntly, I was about as far down as I could get, so why ignore it? I simply acknowledged where I was at that particular time and let it wail. I think it really helped me to let go of it all. I always propped myself up for everyone, including myself. So those rare times when I let myself grieve with really sad music were almost a relief – a way to cleanse my heart and soul. Doing that helped me get back up and find the brighter side of life. It also helped me realize that there are lots of reasons to live. I really did want to stick around on this planet for a while longer.

For every emotion you can feel, someone out there has found a way to put it to music. There's music for meditating, making love, expressing anger, loneliness, joy. You name it and there's music that can move your heart and soul to that very spot like nothing else. Music can consume your entire being. Embrace the wonderful healing power of music. Let music lift you, heal you and express your emotions. If you need to indulge in some sadness, music is a wonderful expression of the depths of your sorrow. Remember though, let it out and let it go. Move on to your higher vibration. Don't let your grief last forever. You are meant to move past it.

I would be wasting my time if I tried to recommend specific music. Music is as personal as each individual. What I do recommend is that you purchase some form of music or sound specifically meant for healing. In addition, find music that lifts you up with positive lyrics or no lyrics at all. When you hear words and music that reinforce your own unique abilities and powers, the sound will send healing energy to your cells and lift your spirits at the same time.

Sound and music have a long history in the role of healing. From the dawn of civilization, sound and music have been used for healing. Studies have shown that music helps to increase serotonin and growth hormone levels while decreasing stress hormones. Music affects blood pressure, circulation, brain activity and lots of other physical and emotional responses. Hospitals use music to calm patients, help manage pain and reduce complications from surgery.

There's lots of information available about the healing power of music and plenty of healing music to choose from. This is an inexpensive way to make great strides in regaining your health. Music has the power to remind you of who you are and what you can accomplish. Let music take you there. Let it take you to that wondrous place of feeling healthy and vibrantly alive.

There is no reason to leave this planet prematurely. You are an amazing being and we all benefit by your being here. You are valuable beyond words. Music can help you recall and reclaim yourself and your health.

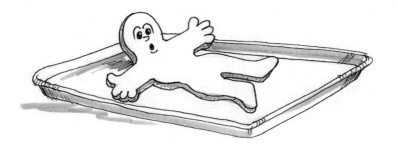

I'm on the Tray

It's true – my photo is "on the tray." You can call me crazy if you like, but I'm not the only one. Thousands of people all over the world are "on the tray." It's all about "energetic balancing."

Everything is energy and everything has a frequency. Everyone and everything vibrates at a unique frequency – even diseases. When you neutralize any energetic imbalances, self-healing can take place. Now, before you jump to any conclusions, please hear me out. I didn't just leap into this without careful thought and study. I had my own doubts and questions about energetic balancing and how it could impact my health.

It all started with Kevin Trudeau's book, *Natural Cures 'They' Don't Want You to Know About*. This led me to read *Sanctuary: The Path to Consciousness*, by Stephen Lewis and Evan Slawson. It's a fascinating book that guided me to EMC² and the spiritual technology of the AIM Program. AIM stands for "All Inclusive Method." It is a system that provides energetic balancing. Participants receive hundreds of thousands of balancing frequencies 24 hours a day, seven days a week, through their photos. Your higher self uses these balancing frequencies to increase your life force and your ability to respond to energetic crises. AIM delivers balancing frequencies for physical and karmic (hereditary) energetic imbalances. It is important to understand that the AIM Program doesn't heal you. Only you can do that. It is a wonderful tool that enables you to heal yourself.

I realize this may sound a little bizarre to you, but it is impossible for me to ignore all the new information from the quantum world. I am learning many new concepts that have to do with quantum physics and quantum holograms. It's confusing and certainly above my intellect. I admit that at the time I enrolled in the AIM Program, I did so mostly based on intuition and what others said about the program. For me it was impossible to ignore people like Dr. Wayne Dyer and Rev. Dr. Michael Beckwith, founder of the Agape International Spiritual Center in Culver City, California. When people with credentials like these talk, I listen! The things they said about AIM and their experiences on the program gave me confidence and reassurance that I'd made a good choice.

I found the EMC² facilitator for my area, Jennifer Hadley, through an Internet search. She directed me to the Agape International Spiritual Center and that's where we met. I met other people on the program, and then Jennifer took my photo and signed me up. Jennifer is an incredible lady. Although she is no longer an EMC² facilitator, she says that she will always remain on the program. She is an awesome writer and a healer in her own right. She seems to radiate spirituality. I look forward to her newsletters and email. Her writing has helped in many areas of my life.

I realize that just because I don't understand how something works, it doesn't mean I can't enjoy its benefits. For example, I don't understand how electricity works, how televisions broadcast pictures or even how my car runs, but I enjoy their benefits. Maybe you feel the same way. The point is that you don't need to understand how or why something works in order to benefit from it.

As you continue to search for new ways to enhance your health, you will find lots of new concepts such as the AIM Program and energetic balancing. I never understood anything about quantum physics. In fact, I'd never even heard of quantum physics until recently, but it's already changed my life. I know it's changed the lives of a lot of people and the way they feel about medicine, particularly the future of medicine. Will we ever see the practice of energetic medicine? Right now, energetic balancing is considered as a spiritual method of self-healing. It isn't practiced conventionally, but maybe some day in the future it will be. Let's face it, you can't ignore what Adam is doing, at least I can't.

I found Adam when I was in the bookstore one day with my friend Dolby, nagging her about drinking more water. As we scanned the books, she opened one right to a section about water! We laughed about that as we moved on to other books. Then, at the same moment, we each picked up a different book by a young man who goes only by the name Adam. We scanned the pages and decided to purchase both books. I'm glad we did.

Adam is a young man from Canada who discovered he could heal people when he was fourteen years old. Not only can he heal people, he's also able to describe how he does it. Guess what? He does it energetically! He describes the quantum hologram, the aura, energy and much more. This amazing young man not only heals people all over the world, he teaches us how to heal ourselves.

Even though I am on the AIM Program, I never understood why energetic balancing doesn't actually heal you, yet it somehow allows you to heal yourself. Now, after reading Adam's books, I understand. Adam explains that after he heals a person energetically, the person must assume responsibility for his or her own healing. The wonderful thing about Adam is his explicit instruction on how to accomplish that healing.

Adam hits the target when it comes to mind, body and spirit. His healings cannot be taken lightly. He has healed people with terminal illnesses such as pancreatic cancer. He clearly explains how his successful healing encompasses the person being healed and that person's willingness to examine every aspect of life. Adam is not only a healer – he is a teacher. I learned so much from his book, *The Path of the DreamHealer*. Lately, I've been buying anything I can get my hands on that Adam has written. His talent and teachings are truly a gift to us all. Do yourself a favor and check out this intelligent, gifted young man's work. Through Adam's teachings, I've expanded the benefits I receive from the AIM Program. He has helped me better understand energetic balancing and my role in the process.

I want to emphasize that you don't have to understand anything about energetic balancing or the AIM Program to benefit from it. Even children benefit from this program. If you don't believe me, you should hear what parents say. The best example is in AIM's outreach program for children with autism and Down syndrome. The improvement in the lives of these children is astounding. When I read the testimonials from their parents, I'm even more grateful for this program. Often after only three months on the program, parents and teachers witness amazing progress in a child's development. You can read some of these testimonials on the web site. In fact, you can learn all about the AIM Program by going to www.energeticmatrix.com.

I encourage you to take a closer look at the crazy world of quantum physics and energetic balancing. Not only will you see changes in your physical heath, you'll find a real mental clarity that comes along with it. I find that I'm able to accomplish many tasks and goals that I never believed possible. I am energized and full of vitality, yet there's a sense of calmness within me. I wish I could better describe my new feeling of wholeness and well-being. Believe me, if there was any way I could eliminate these imbalances on my own, I would. But then again, that would be a full-time job and there are many other things I want to do.

I sincerely believe that there are no coincidences in life. The AIM Program was presented to me for a reason and I made my choice. There are many beautiful enlightened souls out there. I am not one of them. But, I do think I have the ability to sense when I'm in the presence of an enlightened soul. You can feel the genuine love, gratitude and sincerity from these folks as they attempt to make our lives and this world a better place. There are many ways to treat your illness and it's up to you to decide which tools you will use. I like to have lots of tools in my toolbox. But remember, it's up to you to use those tools.

There is always one common thread in all healing practices – and that is you! Remember, the "healing" part is your responsibility. Only you can heal you.

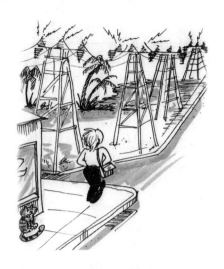

Electromagnetic Frequencies

Some people may say this is a bunch of hogwash, but people who live near towering power lines feel differently. Some feel these power lines bring on diseases such as cancer and arthritis. Often people speak of headaches and a diminished sense of well-being when they're around power lines. But it's not just power lines that generate a hazardous electromagnetic field (EMF). It's cell phones, computers, televisions and all electrical appliances, too.

We are bombarded with so many electromagnetic fields that everyone is affected to some degree. Unfortunately, it's not getting any better. As technology advances, our exposure to EMFs only increases. It's difficult to say exactly what effect this may have on your body, since your body's energy is electrical in nature.

There is such concern over this that in 1996, the World Health Organization (WHO) established the International EMF Project. The way I look at it, if the WHO is concerned, perhaps I should be, too. Luckily, other people are concerned about EMFs and they are doing something about it.

I was relieved to hear that there are ways you can protect yourself. There are products you can purchase for a room, your home and even products to wear. I started with a Q-Link necklace. I wore it constantly. When it didn't go with an outfit I was wearing, I carried it in my pocket or even in my bra. My energy level is higher, yet I feel calmer. I sleep much better, without so many midnight awakenings. My concentration improved as well as my overall sense of well-being. When I bought my Q-Link, I bought one for my husband, too! He wears it every day, under his shirt. I know he feels the benefits or he would have stopped wearing it ages ago. Les is one of those practical guys, not trendy at all. He would be quick to discard it if he didn't feel there was something to it. I'm glad he wears it; after all, he is my love.

Recently I purchased a necklace called Earth Calm. It is quite beautiful. I wear either the Q-Link or the Earth Calm necklace, never both at the same time. Eventually, I plan to get EMF protection for my home. It will be great when everyone who comes into our home is protected.

If you are concerned about this new form of pollution, there's plenty of information out there for you to explore. For me, I know I can't be an expert in every field, so I made the decision based on my own research and findings. As with all things, the decision is yours. I found it to be one of those small things I could do that was pretty much effortless. Why not protect myself? Just because I can't see it, doesn't mean it isn't affecting me. I can't see the radiation that an x-ray emits, but I know it's there. Wearing one of these necklaces is one of those small things you can do to protect your health. It is also one of the easiest. Once you're hooked, you'll get others on board. These are awesome gifts that you can give to anyone. So, start protecting yourself from EMFs. Every little bit helps!

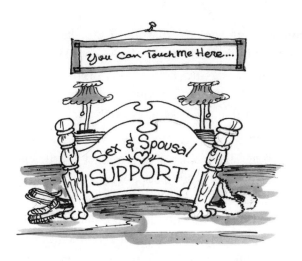

Sex and Spousal Support

When it comes to cancer, most people think only in terms of survival. However, once your cancer treatment becomes routine, you start to wonder if you'll ever have a normal life again. And since sex is part of a "normal" life, it's natural for women to be concerned about it. After all, sex isn't just reserved for the young. As we age, we realize that most people stay sexually active throughout life.

Some of my biggest challenges have been with my feelings about sexuality. I knew I was going to remain sexually active, but how would I cope with all the physical and mental changes that took place in me? My husband and I found ways to be intimate and sexual throughout my treatments, but internally I struggled. I remember the first time we had intercourse after my radical hysterectomy. I was just in so much pain. It wasn't only a lubrication issue. I felt like my vagina was the size of a twelve-year-old child's. It wasn't pleasant, either. I remember being shocked that my doctor hadn't warned me about this. It took a long time before I could handle complete penetration. These issues aren't easily discussed. It is difficult to talk privately with your spouse and doctor about this and it's terribly hard to discuss this publicly.

Although I was sexually active before I joined my support group at The Wellness Community, I still hadn't fully come to terms with how to cope with all the changes. I was surprised when our group leader Joyce suggested that we set aside some time to talk about sex. What surprised me even more was how many women jumped on the topic. Suddenly, everyone wanted to discuss her sexual challenges. What a relief. A few women were astounded to hear that most of us were working very hard to stay sexually active. One woman said she thought her sex life was over because of cancer. Now she realized that most people remain sexually active, cancer or not.

So there it was, out in the open. Sex and cancer became the topic. Believe me, there's plenty to talk about! To start, there are changes in your physical appearance. My new scars aren't exactly appealing. It's difficult to feel sexy when you have so much scarring. We're all somewhat self-conscious when it comes to the way our bodies look, but it's important to get over it, because that's really not the issue. When it comes right down to it, most of our scars and physical changes aren't nearly as ugly as we think they are. Naturally, scars will fade over the years and become less important. I'll admit I do miss my beautiful tummy, mostly for my husband's sake, but it's gone now.

Thank goodness for my wonderful husband with his awesome attitude. He'd rather have me here with a few battle scars than in the grave. He is such a great guy. He's spoiled me ever since I can remember and he hasn't stopped yet. Spousal support makes all the difference when it comes to cancer, healing and sexuality. It's comforting to know that you can still have passionate, intimate and playful sex. But your spouse can only support you if you will allow it. Avoiding sex or the subject of sex isn't going to help either one of you. Talk to each other. If you have fears about sex being safe for you, discuss it with your doctor. Once you've healed from your surgery, there's usually no reason to avoid sex. Resuming sexual activity is good for both of you. The warmth and closeness of sex is reassuring. It keeps you connected and it's fun, too. Sometimes my husband teases me about how hot I get during sex because it often brings on hot flashes. Our little romp in the hay turns into a hunk of burning love in no time!

Hot flashes are common complaint. For years, I had hot flashes daily – almost hourly, in fact. Night sweats are even worse. First, you're burning up as if someone has lit an internal fire. It seems to radiate from within. Anyone who is standing near you can actually feel the heat radiating from you. No kidding! You can't control the sweating. Then, once the hot flash ends, you're left wringing wet and you can actually become chilled. This drives my poor husband crazy, not to mention how miserable it makes me feel. One minute I'm burning up; the next minute I'm freezing! For the most part, my husband jokes about how we now live in the Arctic. My hot flashes have gotten much better over the years, but I still get them occasionally.

It's best to discuss your concerns about hot flashes with your doctor. Lots of things may help. My doctor prefers that

I stay away from any type of hormone treatment and I follow his advice. Hot flashes simply haven't been a priority for me. Don't let my lack of research deter you from seeking out your own remedies. I know many women who have found effective natural solutions for their hot flashes. Lots of ladies swear by Suzanne Somers' recommendations. I haven't tried them, because of the hormone issues. I have to admit that I love her approach to health and diet. Suzanne Somers is another wonderful resource when it comes to healthy lifestyles.

Although I wasn't actively looking for a solution to my hot flashes, I experienced a positive shift in their frequency and intensity when I started the AIM Program in 2003. I didn't expect this as a result of energetic balancing, but it happened! I went from hourly, *raging* hot flashes to maybe a couple each day and that's where it has remained. My hot flashes are easier to manage, too. Often I can avoid the full force of a hot flash by catching it early, drinking cool water or simply fanning myself.

Going through menopause is never easy. I went through menopause overnight because of the radical hysterectomy from ovarian cancer. I didn't think having a hysterectomy would cause hot flashes or any of the other symptoms of menopause. Boy was I wrong! Going through instant menopause causes symptoms far more severe than the slow changes that evolve over time during natural menopause. Menopause really affected my sex drive. I no longer had any of my female internal organs and that became most obvious to me when it came to sex. I understood what women meant when they said they felt like they were an empty shell. It was extremely frustrating. I no longer have natural lubrication in my vagina. Not to mention I felt way too tight. My doctor assured me this would improve over time. He also assured me I could still have orgasms, but I wondered. Even my desire for sex diminished.

With all these changes, I had to learn how to relax and feel sexy again. My sexual desires didn't die out entirely, but they took on a new form. I had to learn about myself all over again. Believe it or not, the best information I received about dealing with cancer and sex came from The Wellness Community. Our support group facilitator gave us booklets from the American Cancer Society titled *Sexuality and Cancer: For the Woman Who Has Cancer and Her Partner*. This little booklet had more straightforward talk about sex than I ever expected. It went into the very things I wanted to ask but was reluctant to discuss in public. The booklet offered solutions to just about every sexual challenge I could think of, from physical to mental. Solutions ranged from self-image to sexual positions. I still have this booklet. I just haven't been able to give it away, as I so often do with my books. It proved such a valuable resource. Of course, I can't ignore the value of our support group discussions that included some very personal and, to some, unthinkable solutions. These were difficult times for all of us, but we were a determined group, working to find ways to overcome our challenges.

Throughout these trying times, I remained sexually active. Most important was the closeness and tenderness I felt with my husband. He was going through as much hell as I was and we both needed to feel loved. I had cancer, but I wasn't dead! It doesn't matter what type of sexual intimacy you choose; it's critical to stay sexually active. I wasn't going to let cancer take away the intimate part of our relationship.

We were both willing to work through the challenges.

Things have changed physically, there's no denying that. My internal sex organs are gone, but they are internal! It doesn't mean I'm not sexually attractive on the outside! I'll admit, it takes time to make adjustments, but it is worth the effort.

Focus on your positive features. When it comes to your physical body, you must stop your negative self-talk. Always remember that you are beautiful just the way you are. Lots of people would feel blessed to make love to you just the way you are, so stop being mean to yourself. You are filled with love and there are many ways to express that love. The simple act of touching is filled with intimacy and it can be very sensual. Caress each other and enjoy the closeness. Make love in new ways if the old way is no longer pleasing. Don't be afraid to discuss sex with your partner and be open to suggestions. Love and intimacy play an essential role in healing.

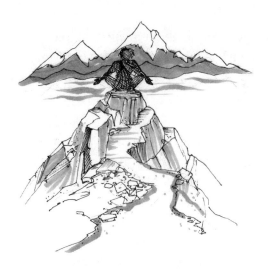

Tall Order for a Spiritual Journey

I've often heard people say, "When you die, that's it. You're dead. There is no more." Usually these are people who aren't personally facing death. They may have experienced the death of a loved one or even witnessed the slow deterioration of a spouse. Many are angry. They question the absence (or presence) of God during their loved one's suffering. For them, there is no spiritual journey – only an end. I believe this type of thinking changes when you find the Grim Reaper looking directly at you. When death approaches slowly, it's like a long rainstorm.

At some point during these stormy times, you will look inward. There's just no avoiding it. Facing the real possibility of death causes you to examine your life, review your accomplishments, judge your behaviors and reflect. It may seem strange to think about a spiritual journey at this time, but isn't that what death is? It's your very own personal journey into the unknown. It is a passage you take, and you take it all by yourself.

Once the dust settles and you no longer need constant care, you'll find that you have a great deal of time to yourself. This time spent alone is different. You're recovering; you are healing. No matter how positive you are in your daily life, this time alone will bring very deep thoughts. This is when you'll evaluate the seriousness of your condition with truth. You'll begin to hold yourself accountable in some way, wondering how you contributed to your current state. You may wonder where God is during this time. I'd grappled with my beliefs about God long before I had cancer and I returned to this subject during my down time. No matter what you believe, you're sure to have questions and doubts. Some of my personal questions may be the same ones you find yourself asking.

I wondered if my life had made a difference. I thought about being only a memory, a photo on someone's wall. What would that be like? What would people say about me? Had I been fair? Had I given people my true self or had I given them who I wanted them to think I was? How genuine had my life been?

I know I've lived a full life. I have more than I dreamed. My youth was full of adventure, risk and fun. Although I'd had plenty of hardships, I recall the richness of my life. My children and grandchildren are another way that my life has been enriched. My husband and I have the relationship we've both always wanted in our marriage. We've traveled to many parts of the world. I couldn't deny the fact that it may very well have been my time to die. I couldn't barter about things I hadn't accomplished. Many people justifiably fall into this category, but not me. I knew it could have been my time.

It helps to know that you've lived a full life, but it's not enough when you're at death's doorstep. It does little to resolve the fear and loneliness you feel. How do you come to terms with the prospect of your physical life coming to an end? I know I'd made compromises during my life. I hoped they were the right ones. Had I followed my true path? I became brutally honest in my self-evaluations. I really wanted to know what was in my soul. Who's inside there? Sometimes, I found myself almost a stranger. I'd try to stare myself down, looking directly through outside eyes. It was uncomfortable, because you look physically different, not bad, but there are subtle differences. I wanted to know the "me" inside me and what I was all about. I didn't want to die without coming to terms with my own spirituality.

Going inward and doing this type of work is very personal. And it will be intensely spiritual. We all are guilty of neglecting ourselves in some manner, particularly when it comes to nurturing our spiritual lives. This is the perfect time to do some necessary spiritual work. You have plenty of time and few distractions. There is much to think about when you are evaluating your life. You may find yourself wanting to talk about some of this with others. It can be helpful to hear another's opinion. While some things are good to talk about, other areas of your spiritual journey are private and could even be considered sacred, particularly if you make the commitment to go deep into your soul.

Conversations between you and your soul, God or whatever you believe will be quite moving. Many call this connecting to Source. This spiritual connection may be the most important part of your healing. A spiritual journey is always humbling. You will be exposing your true self. This is where you learn all about your own private rulebook. Your senseless needs, your false beliefs, your pride, your resentment and your justifications all come to the surface; many are products of your foolish rulebook. There is much to explore – so many pieces, some broken, some missing and some simply well hidden. You must be willing to surrender to honesty and acceptance. You need to be whole again and that's not easy. Even if you feel as though your efforts are not 100 percent successful, remember, intention is all that matters.

When you find yourself this deep into your spiritual journey, it will not be something that you can chat about lightly with friends. This is very private stuff. You will work out the issues of your life in your interior. Your soul is not open for public discussion or debate. The time you spend alone with your thoughts will lead you down many paths. You'll find that you are a deeply complex person. Stick with it; there is healing in your honesty. You will certainly own up to your weaknesses and failures, but at the same time your power and greatness will become illuminated and glorious. You will find your connectedness with all that is, ever was, and ever will be.

You are here now. You are alive. You are on a path.

You'll find many paths that lead to the same place. The path you take is of little importance. It is only important that you follow a spiritual path. You may find your spirituality in a particular religion or it may take another form. There is no right or wrong when it comes to connecting with Source, the universe, God or your soul. It is a journey we all must take alone. No one can go to the interior of your soul except you. It is your path of healing. As you do this, you will discover not only your true self, but also the magnificent gift of living.

Focus on complete healing. That means heal all parts of you. If you don't know where to start your spiritual journey, start it from within. Once you start clearing the debris, your path will become clear to you. Your spiritual journey will be as unique as you are. It is time to heal. You are already working on healing your body; so why not work on healing your mind and soul as well? There is no healing without including your total being. Find the spiritual path that is right for you. Relish it and then embrace your healing.

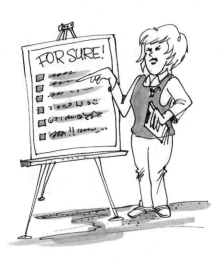

What I Know for Sure

I've always admired Oprah Winfrey. Who doesn't? She is the ultimate role model. She uses her fame and wealth to help others in unimaginable ways. Whether it's financial, moral or spiritual, Oprah shares it all. I believe she is one of those rare souls who are helping to lift the consciousness of humanity.

Oprah often sums up a topic by saying, "Here's what I know for sure." Her catchy phrase had me asking, "What exactly do I know for sure?" I know I've been through hell and back, but what do I know for sure?

Well, one thing I know for sure is that things change all the time. New discoveries are made daily and many of them pertain to our health. As we learn more, old treatments often fall by the wayside – either because they were proven ineffective or because something better came along. This may not always happen. Sometimes old remedies come back with a new twist or renewed enthusiasm, particularly when a new remedy creates more problems than it solves. I have no doubt that there will come a day when we will look back on our current cancer treatments with horror and disbelief. That will be a welcome change. Whether we are surviving because of the current treatment regime or in spite of it, many of us are surviving and that is good.

Whatever the case may be, I continue to do my research and I try new things for my health and continued healing because things change all the time. New information is always available. It's interesting and exciting to read, evaluate and determine what I might try next. Some of the things I've done to achieve heath may end up having no validity at all. Others may prove to be effective beyond current beliefs and open up a completely new realm of healing possibilities. Either way, I don't become attached to the outcome. If a remedy proves useless, then I move on to something else. The main thing is to keep at it. You cannot expect good health if you neglect or poison your body. You must realize that being healthy is an ongoing process. That's another thing I know for sure.

I also know that healing comes in many forms. Conventional medicine, alternative treatments and complementary therapies stand out, but they aren't the only healing tools available. I've learned that miracles still happen – even today.

I've also learned that one belief or form of treatment isn't necessarily going to cure you. Often many things contribute to your healing. Cards, letters, phone calls, gifts and visits all play an important role in your healing. The people who do these things probably don't even realize how much you benefit from their kind and loving gestures. The people in your life have a tremendous impact on your healing.

Although I don't consider myself religious in the traditional sense, I am very spiritual. So when people told me they were praying for me, I welcomed their prayers with gratitude and open arms. Never underestimate the power of prayer. Even when people you don't know pray for you, the benefits are measurable. We all have healing qualities and when we project these healing abilities towards other people, whether through prayer, positive thinking or energy, there is a benefit.

You can enjoy the full benefits of healing when you take a total approach. This means healing your body, your mind and your spirit. Throughout my illness, I felt scattered and fragmented. My thoughts were all over the place. My body was in shambles and my spirit was broken. Slowly, I started the collection process. It was as if I was collecting the shattered pieces of my soul.

At first I didn't know where to look or how to begin, but slowly, one step at a time, I found my way. I began by paying attention to my physical body. As my body got stronger, my mind became clearer. Then I made a conscious effort to use my mind in a positive manner. I worked to control my thinking by being attentive to my thoughts. When I had negative thoughts, I found a way to reword them into something positive. I read health books, stories of spiritual journeys and survivor stories. Collecting the pieces of a life after cancer isn't as simple as it might sound. Reading survivor stories helped reveal some places I hadn't thought to look to as sources for healing. What each person needs to heal is as unique as that individual. While each survivor's story varies, you'll begin to see similarities that can serve as guidance. There are numerous sources for guidance, help and support. You only have to look, seek or ask. This I know for sure.

While it's true that we won't live in these bodies forever, it doesn't mean we have to leave prematurely. The fact that we have cancer doesn't necessarily mean it's our time to go. Although that may be the case, none of us knows for certain. There are many things we don't know for certain. We probably *don't* know more than we *do* know.

What I know for sure about cancer is that it comes with great suffering. Suffering is part of living. We will all suffer in some way or another during our lives. How we deal with that suffering determines the outcome. Fear, worry, dark thoughts and negativity will not help ease your suffering. I had to learn to face my suffering head on and accept it for what it was. It was painful and I felt pitiful and helpless. And then I turned my suffering into appreciation and gratitude. I know this sounds absurd. How could anyone be grateful for cancer? Well, I found a way. I thanked God that I was the one suffering, not one of my daughters or one of my sisters. I had lived a full life and they were young, most with families and much at stake. I found appreciation that cancer had passed them up and settled on me. I accepted my suffering as far more tolerable than seeing any of them go through this torture. I knew the real extent of the suffering and agony – and it took a toll. That made me even more thankful to know it was me, not them. Love and gratitude for them helped me through the suffering. I know for sure that these powerful forces aided my healing.

When it's all said and done, conjuring up a cure is how I get through every day. Finding what works takes time and commitment. I know some people will disregard many of the healing techniques I've embraced. I also know many people don't want to put much effort into healing. Many say they can't make lifestyle changes or they don't believe the changes will make a difference in their health.

Whatever you believe about healing and health, keep in mind that your doctor can only treat your disease. Your doctor cannot maintain your good health for you. Only you can do that. It is up to you.

The great thing about being healthy after a life-threatening disease is the joy of living your new life to the fullest. Your lifestyle changes become fun and effortless. Each morning becomes another good morning and each moment becomes the only one that counts. Before you realize it, you are living a joyous life full of appreciation, gratitude and love. Conversations no longer include cancer and life takes on new purpose and meaning. It is exhilarating and wonderful.

The best part of being healthy (and possibly the most dangerous part) is that you can afford to be a little reckless now and then. You may find yourself willing to take on exciting challenges that you would have avoided prior to your illness. It might be something outrageous such as skydiving or perhaps something as small having a couple of cocktails at a party. I'm not talking about living a reckless life, but living a *chosen* life – a life where an occasional risk or wildness actually feeds your life force.

Fill your life with joy and laughter – and I mean real laughter, the kind that makes your belly ache and eyes tear. I recall the many times laughter helped me, even as tears of despair poured down my face. The healing quality of laughter has been studied and it is well documented. You always feel better when you are laughing, even if it is painful at the time. This is another thing I know for sure.

What I know for sure is not always easy to define, especially when it comes to ovarian cancer. My thoughts keep returning to one of my favorite t-shirts. It's a John Lennon t-shirt. The front displays a small piece of his artwork (a little guy looking through a camera). The back of the t-shirt shows a large picture of John. It's what he said on the t-shirt that really strikes a chord with me. The t-shirt reads, "The more I see, the less I know for sure." That pretty much sums up my feelings when it comes to what I know for sure. My knee-jerk reaction is to say, "I don't know anything for sure!" But that simply isn't true.

Here is what I know for sure. Life's challenges are rarely easy. Cancer and other life-threatening diseases can be overcome. You *can* heal yourself and the time to start is now. There is no other time. There is only the present moment. And most important of all, please know that you are not alone.

References Cited and My Personal Recommendations

Books

- *A Course in Miracles*, by Dr. Helen Schucman and published by the Foundation for Inner Peace. Expect miracles, but you must be dedicated to complete this course because it takes a year to do the workbook exercises.

- *A Guide to Survivorship for Women with Ovarian Cancer,* by F.J., Montz MD, K.M., FACOG, FACS and Robert E. Bristow, MD, FACOG.

- *A Life of Miracles*, by Almine. A great spiritual read.

- *A New Earth*, by Eckhart Tolle. A must-read. Transform your consciousness and awaken to your inner life's purpose.

- *Alkalize or Die*, by Dr. Theodore A. Baroody.

- *Anatomy of an Illness*, by Norman Cousins. Learn to use humor to heal and not take life too seriously.

- *Ask and It Is Given*, by Esther and Jerry Hicks. This is one of my favorites. Learn to manifest your healing desires.

- *Beating Cancer with Nutrition*, by Patrick Quillin PhD, RD, CNS.

- *Cure for All Advanced Cancers*, by Hulda Regehr Clark, PhD, ND.

- *Cure for All Cancers*, by Hulda Regehr Clark, PhD, ND.

- *Cure for All Diseases*, by Hulda Regehr Clark, PhD, ND.

- *Disappearance of the Universe*, by Gary R. Renard. Straight talk about illusions, past lives, religion, sex, politics and the miracles of forgiveness.

- *DreamHealer: A True Story of Miracle Healings*, by Adam. Powerful teachings on the effect our beliefs and expectations have on our health.

- *Entering the Castle*, by Caroline Myss. An intense soulful journey leading to the path of God.

- *Healing with the Angels*, by Doreen Virtue, PhD. We all have angels. Learn how to call on them to assist you.

- *Hidden Messages in Water*, by Masaru Emoto. See how thoughts, intentions and words change water and the impact this has on your body.

- *How to Practice*, by His Holiness, the Dalai Lama.

- *It's All In Your Head*, by Dr. Hal A. Huggins. Explains the link between mercury amalgams (dental fillings) and illness.

- *It's Not About the Bike*, by Lance Armstrong.

- *Natural Cures 'They' Don't Want You to Know About*, by Kevin Trudeau. Learn about processed, manipulated and engineered food products. Here's where I learned that drugs, labels and ingredients aren't what they appear to be.

- *Path of the DreamHealer*, by Adam. Adam is an energy healer who teaches us how to use quantum physics to heal ourselves.

- *Places That Scare You*, by Pema Chödrön. A guide to fearlessness in difficult times.

- *Power of Now*, by Eckhart Tolle.

- *Profound Healing*, by Cheryl Canfield.

- *Sacred Contracts*, by Caroline Myss.

- *Sanctuary*, by Stephen Lewis and Evan Slawson. Learn about the spiritual practice of energetic balancing to heal yourself.

- *Sexuality & Cancer*, an American Cancer Society publication.

- *The Cancer Cure That Worked*, by Barry Lynes. Discovery and suppression of the cancer cure that worked.

- *The Five People You Meet in Heaven*, by Mitch Albom.

- *The pH Miracle*, by Robert O. Young, PhD, and Shelly Redford Young. Learn how to balance your body's pH for optimal health.

- *The Patient Active Guide to Living with Ovarian Cancer*, by The Wellness Community – National.

- *The Secret*, by Rhonda Byrne. How to manifest everything you've ever wanted.

- *The Sexy Years*, by Suzanne Somers. Discover natural bioidentical hormone replacement therapy.

- *Tooth Truth*, by Frank J. Jerome, DDS. If you want to be healthy, don't metal with your teeth.
- *True Power of Water*, by Masaru Emoto.
- *When Things Fall Apart*, by Pema Chödrön. Advice that actually helps in difficult times.
- *You Can Heal Your Life*, by Louise Hay. What we think about ourselves becomes the truth for us.

CDs
- *Awakening Prologue*, by Holosync Solution
- *Chakra Clearing*, by Doreen Virtue
- *Change Your Thoughts – Change Your Life*, by Dr. Wayne Dyer
- *Dark Side of the Light Chasers*, by Debbie Ford
- *Don't Bite the Hook*, by Pema Chödrön
- *Entering the Castle*, by Caroline Myss
- *Getting Ready*, by Bernie S. Siegel, MD
- *Meditations for Enhancing Your Immune System*, by Bernie S. Siegel, MD
- *Personal Healing*, by Caroline Myss
- *Power to Create*, by Caroline Myss
- *Self Esteem*, by Caroline Myss
- *The Key*, by Joe Vitale
- *Sanctuary*, by Stephen Lewis and Evan Slawson
- *You Are What You Love*, by Vaishali
- *You Staying Young*, by Michael F. Roizen, MD and Mehment C. Oz, MD

DVDs
- *Cancer Doesn't Scare Me Anymore*, by Lorraine Day, MD
- *Change Your Thoughts, Change Your Life*, by Dr. Wayne Dyer
- *DreamHealer: Visualizations for Self-Empowerment*, by Adam
- *The Secret*, Rhonda Byrne, Jack Canfield, Neale Donald Walsch and Others

- *There's a Spiritual Solution to Every Problem*, by Dr. Wayne Dyer
- *You Can Heal Your Life*, by Louise Hay
- *You Can't Improve On God*, by Lorraine Day, MD
- *What the Bleep!? – Down the Rabbit Hole*, Directed by Mark Vicente, Betsy Chasse, William Arntz

Web Sites

www.cancer.org – American Cancer Society

www.drclarkstore.com – Resources for Dr. Clark's treatment recommendations

www.drclarkuniversity.org – Healing products and information

www.drday.com – Dr. Lorraine Day's web site

www.dreamhealer.com – Adam

www.energeticmatrix.com – Sanctuary and AIM Program for energetic balancing

www.healingmusic.org – The Healing Music Foundation

www.immunotec.com – Immunocal web site

www.lifesourcewater.com – Carbon filtration water systems

www.miraculewater.com/Distilledwater.php – Learn about water

www.mysticsoulscafe.com – Support group, products, books

www.naturalcures.com – Alternatives to drugs and surgery

www.ovariancancer.org – Ovarian Cancer National Alliance

www.triangularwave.com – Why soft water is not for drinking

www.wellnesscommunity.org – Support group